Improving Sexual Health Advice

Gill Wakley
Freelance General Practitioner
Visiting Professor
Centre for Health Policy and Practice
Staffordshire University

Margaret Cunnion
Senior Lecturer
Staffordshire University

and

Ruth Chambers
General Practitioner
Professor of Primary Care Development
Staffordshire University
Head of Stoke-on-Trent Teaching PCT Programme

Dear Chris

Hope you find this useful

Mary (Cunnion

Cunnion).

Radcliffe Medical Press

Radcliffe Medical Press Ltd
18 Marcham Road
Abingdon
Oxon OX14 1AA
United Kingdom

www.radcliffe-oxford.com
The Radcliffe Medical Press electronic catalogue and online ordering facility.
Direct sales to anywhere in the world.

British Library Cataloguing in Publication Data

A catalogue record for this book is available from the British Library.

ISBN 1 85775 803 X

Typeset by Aarontype Ltd, Easton, Bristol
Printed and bound by TJ International Ltd, Padstow, Cornwall

Contents

Acknowledgements

We developed the contents of this book in conjunction with a range of educational initiatives aimed at reducing teenage pregnancy rates. Gina Milsom developed the learning needs questionnaire, included in Chapter 2, whilst funded by Staffordshire University. Kate Ryan worked with Margaret Cunnion on the sexual health needs assessment described in Chapter 3. We are very grateful for the substantial help and guidance in evolving the format of the learning needs assessment from Mr John Howard and Professor Alan Gillies of the University of Central Lancashire. The Staffordshire County Teenage Pregnancy Steering Group sponsored a series of multi-agency sexual health training workshops, into which the training needs analysis fed, and from which this book was developed.

About the authors

Gill Wakley MB ChB MD MFFP MIPM
Gill started in general practice but transferred shortly afterwards into community medicine and then into public health. A desire for increased contact with patients caused a move back into general practice, together with community gynaecology. She has been combining the two in varying amounts ever since. Throughout she has been heavily involved in learning and teaching. She was in a training general practice, became a Member of the Faculty of Family Planning and Reproductive Health Care and a Member of the Institute of Psychosexual Medicine. She was until recently a senior clinical lecturer with the Primary Care Department at Keele University and is now a visiting professor at Staffordshire University in the Centre for Health Policy and Practice. Like Ruth, she has run all types of educational initiatives and activities. Now partially retired, she combines writing and lecturing with part-time work as a freelance GP.

Margaret Cunnion BSc (Hons) RN Dip HE
Margaret is a staff nurse/health advisor within genito-urinary medicine and a senior lecturer at Staffordshire University. Her clinical experience has made her aware of the urgent need to educate young people in safer sexual practices. Young clinic attendees appeared to be completely unaware of the many sexually transmitted infections other than HIV that have no cure and are prevalent in the community. Margaret is currently managing a sexual health needs assessment of young people within South Staffordshire. She is coordinating a series of multi-agency sexual health training courses for health and social care professionals and others with responsibility for young people. Margaret has a specific interest in young people with special educational needs and has founded a parent support group in Uttoxeter.

Ruth Chambers BM BS DM FRCGP; ruthchambers.com
Ruth has been a general practitioner for more than 20 years. She is the head of the Stoke-on-Trent Teaching Primary Care Trust programme and the national education lead for the NHS Alliance. She is currently the Professor of Primary Care Development at the Centre for Health Policy and Practice at Staffordshire University. Ruth is a member of the Children's Taskforce in England and co-chair of one of the seven external working groups within the Children and Young People's National Service Framework. Over the last five years or so,

Ruth has become increasingly involved with educational and service-based projects to reduce teenage conception rates. Young people have been involved as an integral part of all these initiatives. Ruth has published widely on sexual health through books co-authored with Gill and research reports.

Glossary

Abortion	The ending of a pregnancy either by miscarriage or a termination of pregnancy.
Abstinence	Not having any sexual intercourse.
AIDS	Acquired immune deficiency syndrome. This illness is caused by the human immunodeficiency virus (HIV). It is spread from one person to another by unprotected sex or by injecting drugs with dirty (infected) needles. In most countries blood for transfusion is tested for this infection before a transfusion is given, but this was not the case when the infection was first discovered. A person can have HIV for many years without knowing it.
Antenatal	The period between getting pregnant and having the baby.
Bacterial vaginosis (BV)	When the vagina contains lots of bacteria that do not like much oxygen (anaerobic). It is often associated with getting soap or detergents in the vagina. It can cause a minor irritation that increases the flow of mucus and can produce an unpleasant fishy smell. (See Sexually transmitted infections.)
Barrier methods	The use of condoms, caps or diaphragms to prevent the sperm from reaching the egg.
Candida	A type of fungus (thrush or monilia) that can grow on various parts of the body, including the mouth and vagina.
Cap	A small, latex, dome-shaped device that fits over the cervix. It is usually used to hold a spermicide cream or jelly next to the cervix to inactivate the sperm.
Cervical smear (smear)	A thin film of cells taken from the end of the cervix is spread on a glass slide for examination under a microscope. It is taken to look for early signs of cells that might grow into cancer cells several years later. It sometimes picks up signs of infection as well.
Cervix	The neck of the womb. The narrow end of the uterus that projects into the upper part of the vagina.
Chlamydia	An infection common in young people that can sometimes cause severe problems such as pelvic infection and infertility. Most people do not have any symptoms or

	signs of the infection. It can stay dormant for months or years. (See Sexually transmitted infection.)
Clitoris	A part of the female genitals positioned in front of the vagina and urethra. It is a small, very sensitive, projection of an organ, which becomes filled with blood on stimulation. It can vary in size and can be covered by a hood to a greater or lesser degree. The rest of the erectile tissue in the woman is hidden behind the clitoris and lies around the urethra and front wall of the vagina.
Coitus interruptus	Pulling out the penis before ejaculation. A risky method of contraception.
Colposcopy	Examination of the cervix with a high-powered lens. The cervix is usually painted with diluted acetic acid (purified diluted vinegar) to show up any areas of inflammation.
Combined oral contraceptive (COC)	Combined oral contraceptive containing both oestrogen and progesterone. Used to prevent pregnancy.
Conception	The fertilisation of the woman's egg by the man's sperm.
Condom	A sheath of latex or polyurethane that covers the penis during sexual intercourse to reduce the chances of infection and pregnancy. Female polyurethane condoms, that cover part of the vulva and line the vagina, are also available.
Contraception	The prevention of unwanted pregnancy. Methods of contraception are barriers, pills, intrauterine devices, injections, implants and sterilisation – see individual entries.
Crabs (body lice)	See sexually transmitted infection.
Cystitis	Inflammation of the urinary bladder caused by infection. It can be triggered by sexual intercourse, not drinking enough fluids and poor hygiene.
Delivery	When the baby is born.
Diaphragm	A method of contraception consisting of a dome-shaped piece of latex, which fits across the top of the vagina to hold spermicide against the cervix. It helps to prevent the sperm from entering the uterus.
Ejaculation	When the semen (the liquid carrying sperm) squirts out of the penis.
Embryo	The fertilised egg at the beginning of pregnancy in the early stages of its development. At the beginning of the third month of pregnancy the name of the developing egg is changed to fetus (sometimes spelt foetus and pronounced feet-us).

Emergency contraception	Used after unprotected sexual intercourse or when the method of contraception has failed. The pill method needs to be taken as soon as possible and definitely within 72 hours. The intrauterine device can be fitted within five days of the calculated ovulation date. (See Contraception.)
Endometrium	The lining of the womb or uterus.
Episiotomy	A cut made in the vulva and lower part of the vagina to enlarge the opening through which a baby is born. After delivery it is repaired by stitching.
Erection	When the penis becomes stiff. The penis is made of special tissue called erectile tissue, which acts like a sponge. When the tissue fills with blood, the penis becomes large and erect. Erections occur when the tissue is stimulated by emotions or friction. Even small babies have erections.
Fallopian tubes	Tubes which lead from the ovary to the womb or uterus. The muscular walls can push the egg down to the uterus.
Family planning clinic	Family planning clinics offer a range of services paid for by the National Health Service, so that they are free to the user. Services available include contraception (including condoms), pregnancy testing, cervical screening and advice. The doctors and nurses are specially trained and will have all the latest information. Patients may take a partner or friend if they wish. The service is completely confidential.
Fetus/foetus	An unborn child from three months until it is born.
Foreskin	The end of the penis is covered by a loose fold of skin to protect it. Some boys have an operation called circumcision to remove the foreskin.
Genital herpes	The herpes virus can cause single cold sores or several small sores on the sexual organs or elsewhere. The first attack is often very painful. The virus is spread by contact with a sore, but sometimes the virus can be present on the skin before the sore appears. At present there is no cure but symptoms can be helped with treatment. (See Sexually transmitted infection.)
Genito-urinary medicine	The genito-urinary medicine (GUM) clinic offers a range of services paid for by the National Health Service, so that they are free to the user. All treatment is free, including all prescriptions, and the clinic will pay all reasonable travelling expenses. Services available include full genital testing, emergency contraception, condoms, pregnancy testing, cervical screening and advice. The doctors

and nurses are specially trained and have the latest information available. Patients can just ring up and make an appointment; they do not have to be referred by their doctor. They may take a partner or friend if they wish. The service is completely confidential. All patient records at the GUM clinic are completely separate from all other medical records, including GP and hospital records.

Glans — The rounded sensitive end of the penis.

Gonococcus (GC) — A sexually transmitted disease passed on by vaginal or oral sex. It typically causes symptoms like cystitis or an increase in discharge from the vagina or penis. The infection can be carried without producing any symptoms, especially in women. (See Sexually transmitted infection.)

GP services — Most general practitioners (GPs) offer contraceptive advice, pregnancy testing and cervical smears. GPs must keep the reason that the patient went to see them confidential. Patients can choose to see another doctor for contraceptive advice if they wish. In some practices the nurses may be able to help. Most practices do not give free condoms.

Gynaecologist — A doctor specialising in diseases of women's reproductive organs and adjacent organs such as the urinary tract. Gynaecological complaints refer to problems with the women's reproductive organs.

Haemorrhage — Bleeding heavily.

Homosexuality — Sexual attraction or activity between two people of the same sex.

Human papilloma virus (HPV) — A large number of these viruses have been identified. They can cause warts but infections are not always visible. A few varieties of the virus have been shown to be associated with a greater risk of cancer of the cervix, but can be picked up early by regular cervical smears.

Hymen — A fold of skin covering part, or all, of the opening to the vagina at birth. It often stretches or is broken when being active and when using tampons. Sometimes enough remains across the opening to be broken when having sex for the first time. The fold of skin can bleed when it is broken.

Implant — A plastic tube containing a hormone, usually referring to one to prevent pregnancy. It is put under the skin and releases the hormone slowly.

Incidence — The rate of occurrence of *new* episodes of that illness or characteristic being measured in a sample or population.

Infertility	When a woman cannot get pregnant.
Injection	Usually referring to a contraceptive injection containing a progesterone hormone.
Intrauterine device (IUD)	A small plastic and copper tube put inside the woman's uterus (womb) to prevent pregnancy. (See Contraception.)
Intrauterine system (IUS)	An intrauterine device that has a hormone delivery system. (See Contraception.)
Labia	Sometimes called lips. Folds of skin on the outside of the vulva area around the opening to the vagina. They can be many different shapes and sizes from almost flat to long and dangly. There are two sets. The outside ones are called the labia majora, the inside ones the labia minora.
Labour	Giving birth to a baby.
Laparoscopy	The use of a fine, flexible light tube to inspect organs or treat conditions inside a body cavity.
Masturbation	Stimulating the sexual organs, especially one's own, by means other than sexual intercourse.
Menarche	The first-ever monthly period.
Menstrual	Anything to do with a woman's monthly period.
Miscarriage	The expulsion from the uterus of a fetus that is not developing. Also called a spontaneous abortion.
Morning-after pill	See Emergency contraception.
Mucus	The protective lubricant coating produced by glands. Mucus keeps surfaces like the walls of the vagina moist.
Non-specific urethritis (NSU)	Swelling and soreness of the urethra (the tube which carries urine) caused by infections. (See Sexually transmitted infection.)
Obstetrician	A doctor who specialises in pregnancy and childbirth.
Oestrogen/estrogen	One of the hormones produced by the ovary and responsible for female sexual characteristics. Together with progesterone it causes the changes that occur during a menstrual cycle (monthly). It is one of the hormones in the combined oral contraceptive pill.
Oral sex	When one partner uses the mouth or tongue to stimulate the sexual sensitive parts of another person.
Orgasm	The climax of sexual excitement. Sometimes called 'come' when the man ejaculates semen. The blood in erectile tissue is usually released after the orgasm and the sexual organs become flatter and less erect.
Ovary/ovaries	Women have two ovaries that lie low down in the female abdomen and produce the female hormones and eggs. They are about the size of an almond nut.

Ovulation	When the egg is released from the ovary and starts its journey down the fallopian tube to the uterus.
Ovum	The egg produced in the ovaries before fertilisation.
Paediatrician	A doctor who treats children.
Penis	The man's sexual organ. Penises vary in size and can be anything from 3.5–10 cm long when limp and 9–20 cm when erect. Like other parts of the body, it does not matter how big it is, just how well it works.
Pills	Usually refers to hormones given as a contraceptive.
Placenta	A flat plate of tissue attached to a baby by a cord at one end and the woman's uterus at the other. It acts as a link between the mother's blood supply and the baby. It carries food, oxygen and antibodies.
Planning a pregnancy	There is no set time to have a child. The right time is when the couple feel able to take on all the responsibilities of a child. It makes sense to plan a pregnancy for two reasons: 1 having a child changes the mother's life for ever 2 preparing for a pregnancy means a higher chance of a healthy baby.
Prevalence	The proportion of people in a sample that have that characteristic or illness. (See Incidence.)
Progestogen-only pill (POP)	A pill containing only one of the hormones produced by the ovary. Used to prevent pregnancy.
Puberty	The stage in early adolescence when the individual becomes capable of sexual reproduction and the sexual characteristics appear.
Pubic lice	Tiny insects that are spread from one body to another by contact with someone who has them. (See Sexually transmitted infection.)
Rubbers	Another of the many names for condoms.
Safe sex	Having sex in a way that cuts down the chance of catching a sexually transmitted infection. This includes using a condom.
Scrotum	The sac or bag of skin which hangs down at the back of the penis. Each side contains a testis. It is outside of the body to help keep the testis at the right temperature for the sperm to be active.
Semen	Creamy, sticky fluid produced in the male organs to carry the sperm, which is forcefully released from the penis during sexual activity.
Sexual intercourse	Genital stimulation usually including the insertion of the penis into the vagina.

Sexually transmitted disease (STD)/ sexually transmitted infection (STI)	Infection spread from one person to another through direct body contact or close contact with body fluids. The terms are used to describe infections usually spread by sexual contact.
Sheath	See Condom.
Spermicide	A cream or jelly containing a chemical to help prevent sperm from fertilising eggs. The chemical works better in the test tube than when mixed with mucus in the vagina.
Sterilisation	The removal of the chance of infection from materials such as instruments OR A method of contraception that involves cutting, tying, sealing or putting a clip on the tubes carrying the egg or the sperm. In men it is called vasectomy.
Termination of pregnancy (TOP)	An operation or insertion of instruments and/or drugs to remove an embryo or fetus from the uterus. In the UK this can only be done under strict legal restrictions.
Testicles	Another name for the testes.
Testis/testes (plural)	A male has two testes, each the size of a plum, that lie in the scrotum. The testis produces sperm and the male hormone testosterone.
Testosterone	A male hormone which is responsible for the changes at puberty such as voice changes and facial hair.
Thrush	Information about thrush is in the chapter on STIs although it is not usually sexually transmitted. It is a fungus that causes inflammation, soreness and itching. (See Candida.)
Trichomonas vaginitis (TV)	An infection of the vagina or the urethra that is caused by a tiny parasite. It is usually sexually transmitted but can be found in moist, warm atmospheres such as Jacuzzis and steam rooms. (See Sexually transmitted infection.)
Trimester	Pregnancy is divided into three trimesters: the first trimester until 12 weeks, the second from 13 to 18 weeks and the third from 19 weeks until delivery.
Urethra	The tube that leads down from the bladder to the outside of the body. It also takes the semen to the outside.
Uterus	Often known as the womb. A pear-shaped female organ about 8 cm long. It holds the fetus while it is developing. The muscular walls push out the fetus at delivery.
Vagina	The vagina is the passage leading from the outside of a woman's body to the uterus inside the body. Strong muscles surround the lower third of the vagina. It is soft,

	moist and stretchy to allow the penis to enter and a baby be born through it.
Vasectomy	See Sterilisation.
Venereal disease (VD)	Another name for sexually transmitted disease or infection.
Virgin	A person who has not had sex.
Vulva	The woman's external genitals consisting of the labia, the clitoris and the opening to the vagina called the vestibule.
Warts	Warts are caused by human papilloma viruses. They can occur on any part of the body, including the genitals. (See Sexually transmitted infection.)
Withdrawal	A risky method of contraception that involves taking the penis out of the vagina before ejaculation.
Womb	See Uterus.

Introduction

How you use this book depends on *you*. Successful continuing professional development, education and training relies on focusing on *your* specific and identified needs. Most of us in the past learnt about things that interested us most. Some of the time we learnt about things that did not interest us much, but the learning opportunity turned up and was connected with some other sort of reward such as a good meal, a certificate or promotion and extra monetary reward. Now we need to focus our learning onto the things that we really need to learn. Time is too short and opportunities too precious for us to be unfocused and we must target our learning more effectively.

You have identified that you need to learn more about sexual health – but what do you need to know? The start of any learning activity is to establish what you know already, determine what you need to know by the end, and, hey presto – the gap in the middle is what you need to learn about. You will be able to apply your new learning to meet the sexual health needs in the population and improve the care received in the service in which you work.

You might want to start by reading the first chapter to find out what has changed about the aspirations for the provision of sexual health in primary care and beyond. What is it about a sexual health strategy action plan that is different, possibly even better, than what you and your colleagues were doing before? How can you and your team cater for all these proposals? What information do you need, and what do you need to provide, to improve the management of sexual health in the future? Chapter 1 looks at the challenge of improving sexual health services. It summarises and comments on the *National Strategy for Sexual Health and HIV* for England. It gives you information about the implementation plan for the strategy. Those of you in Scotland, Wales and Northern Ireland have local strategies in place and regional strategies that will be very similar. Other countries have slightly different priorities and plans depending on the sexual health needs of the population. All of this will inform you about what needs to be done in your working environment from the wider perspective of national and regional priorities. It will provide you with the information you need to start to bring together the networks and for clinical governance in sexual health provision.

The requirements that you identify from Chapter 1 include not only your own personal learning needs but also those of colleagues and the changes needed in service provision. The information in Chapter 1 can shape your own personal learning needs but not identify them specifically. Your own experience, reflection and questioning goes a long way towards a more precise evaluation of what you need to learn. In addition to this, Chapter 2 includes information about how you might look at how you learn, as well as how to develop your own skills and knowledge and reflect on your attitudes.

Chapter 2 uses a self-assessment learning needs questionnaire to help you to assess the level at which you are now, and estimate where you need to be in the future. Maximise this self-assessment so as to augment the information from patients, colleagues and managers about what you need to learn. Aim to meet the learning needs that you have identified in order to become competent in what you will be doing in the foreseeable future. We use the term 'competence' to mean the 'ability to perform the tasks and roles required to the expected standard'. Chapter 2 explains how to look at competence, how you might assess your own level of competence and from where you might seek corroborative evidence for your own learning needs assessment.

Competencies are based on an analysis of the professional role and the responsibilities of that role. You already have core competencies in your usual role as a health professional in your particular discipline at a certain level of seniority. You also need knowledge and skills (and suitable attitudes) in sexual health matters on top of those basic competencies. Statements about competencies describe outcomes expected of professionally related activities, or of the knowledge, skills and attitudes thought to be essential to the performance of those activities. A statement about the level of competency required for an activity facilitates the assessment of that activity. It provides a standard that can be compared between individuals. Regard competencies as possible predictors of professional effectiveness but check frequently that the competencies are still valid and accurate. Specify measures and standards for your competencies so that they are capable of being demonstrated publicly and can be accounted for within the framework of clinical governance.

Chapter 2 provides tools for reflecting on, defining and establishing your competencies. The self-assessment questionnaire results in defining the stage (from 1–3) at which you might need to target learning so that you can provide sexual health services. This will be mainly within levels 1 and 2 of the *National Strategy for Sexual Health and HIV*, or the equivalent in countries other than England. Your stage of learning will vary according to your role and required competencies in providing sexual health services or your role and responsibilities in the services you plan to provide.

So you might want to start with Chapter 2, so that you know what you personally need to draw out from Chapter 1 about future provision for sexual health services.

On the other hand, you might want to start by finding out how to do a sexual health needs assessment as detailed in Chapter 3. Without this needs assessment, how can you know what is needed in your region or area? The *National Strategy for Sexual Health and HIV* gives a broad-brush approach, but how will you know what parts are most important for the patients and public in your area without a needs assessment? This measurement underlies all of the provision of health services, for, without knowing what is needed, you cannot begin to evaluate what progress you are making towards meeting those needs. It is no good providing all sorts of services that no one wants, needs or is going to use! On the other hand, you might not provide services that are badly needed or not provide enough of them. So you might want to start with Chapter 3 to identify what is needed in your particular area – but you cannot do this without understanding what is in Chapter 1, and you cannot focus on what you, personally, need in the way of specific competency without working through Chapter 2. Perhaps you had better read them all simultaneously!

So, the first three chapters will help you to focus on your own specific and personal learning needs to establish the level of competency that you require in your role, now and in the immediate future. The chapters that follow provide you with the basic tools to learn about various areas within the broad subject of sexual health. Suggestions are included for further reading so that those who need to become expert or wish to discover more can do so. Embedded within the chapters are icons drawing attention to cultural or religious aspects, together with information about confidentiality, relationships and self-esteem. Chapter 4 on taking a sexual history and Chapter 5 on sexual health screening and investigation underpin these remaining chapters. The chapters on contraception, sexually transmitted infections, more about men, pregnancy and sexual violence could be worked through in the order you prefer. The Appendix provides you with many resources for learning, and access to websites and helplines, that will be of assistance not just with this learning task but also with your future personal development and educational needs.

What is the *National Strategy for Sexual Health and HIV* and what has it to do with me?

What is sexual health?

Sexual health is an important health issue that affects most, if not all, of the population. A large proportion of women will use contraception at some point in their lives and most people have sexual intercourse at some time. Large numbers of people contract sexually transmitted infections (STIs) and rates of STIs in young people in the United Kingdom (UK) are increasing. The UK has the highest teenage pregnancy rates in Western Europe.

A concise and often quoted definition of sexual health is 'enjoyment of the sexual activity of one's choice, without causing or experiencing physical or emotional harm'.[1]

The *Health of the Nation: A strategy for health for England*[2] defined sexual health as:

> Being free, and remaining free from, sexually transmitted diseases and other disorders that can affect reproductive health. Being in control of fertility and avoiding unintended pregnancies. Being able to behave in a sexual way.

In 1975 the World Health Organization (WHO)[3] published a definition of sexual health:

> Sexual health is the integration of the somatic, emotional, intellectual and social aspects of sexual being, in ways that are positively enriching and that enhance personality, communication and love.

In addition the authors included:[3]

> Freedom from fear, shame, guilt, false beliefs and other psychological factors inhibiting sexual responses. Freedom from organic disorder, diseases and deficiencies that interfere with sexual reproductive functions.

Box 1.1 Culture shock

A report in *New Scientist*[5] discusses the way in which the worryingly high and growing number of monogamous, married women testing positive for human immunodeficiency virus (HIV) in their first pregnancy is making people question the professed moral and cultural values in Indian society.

When the number of HIV-positive people in Europe and America was increasing rapidly in the mid-1980s, India believed that it would be protected by its traditional values from a disease spread by sexual promiscuity, prostitution and drug abuse. As in many other countries, India is finding that what appears on the surface of society belies the amount of extramarital and premarital sexual activity hidden by a reluctance to talk about sexual activity openly. Denial of the sexual activity and the risks of catching HIV, together with widespread ignorance and the lower cultural status of women, make combating the spread of HIV more difficult.

The core features of sexual health imply reproductive health, absence of sexual illnesses or disorders, psychosexual well-being and beneficial social interactions. This holistic vision fits into the whole-body medicine concept of primary care.

Paragraph 1.2 of the *National Strategy for Sexual Health and HIV*[4] gives a rather narrower definition and states that:

> Sexual health is an important part of physical and mental health. It is a key part of our identity as human beings together with the fundamental human rights to privacy, a family life and living free from discrimination. Essential elements of good sexual health are equitable relationships and sexual fulfilment with access to information and services to avoid the risk of unintended pregnancy, illness or disease.

This definition medicalises sexual health as a separate 'part of physical and mental health', rather than a holistic facet of human identity and health, perhaps reflecting the interests of those writing the Strategy. This encourages thinking that ignores the wider sociological and cultural environment within which sexual activity occurs and places the emphasis on medical solutions rather than social changes (see Box 1.1).

National Strategy for Sexual Health and HIV

The first *National Strategy for Sexual Health and HIV*[4] was published at the end of July 2001 after the collection of much opinion and evidence. The highlights of the Strategy are:

- a national information campaign aimed at the general public to cover the prevention of STIs, HIV and unintended pregnancies
- a model for sexual health services delivered by every primary care trust that gives nurses and other primary care staff a wider role
- new one-stop sexual health services, which will be piloted and evaluated
- targeted screening for chlamydia
- routine HIV testing in all sexual health clinics
- targets to reduce new infections of HIV and gonorrhoea
- more people offered hepatitis B immunisation in sexual health clinics
- local stakeholders to review sexual health and HIV provision in each area.

Evidence from other countries in Europe shows a link between the culture of open discussion of sexual activity and lower rates of teenage pregnancy and STIs.[6] Whether a national campaign is sufficient to change cultural attitudes in the UK is doubtful. 'No sex, please, we're British' still has too much of a ring of truth. Health promotion departments, and the work being done by many governmental and voluntary bodies, continue to try and raise the profile and level of discussion of sexual health (see Box 1.2).

Specialist health promotion services are run on a shoestring compared, for example, to the amount of money spent by advertisers linking sexuality to their products in an unrealistic, unhealthy way. Film and television dramas portray sexual activity in unrepresentative ways; for example, condoms do not appear in the soap dramas. Without cultural and social change it seems unlikely that more than minor gains will be made by medical efforts alone. Funding by the public information campaign (see Box 1.2) is also being used to provide public information on STIs. Leaflets on common infections that are written in clear language, and have been tested on the target population to ensure that they are understood, are a useful resource for health professionals as well (see Box 1.3). In some areas supplies of the leaflets are available from the health education departments' budgets. In others they will have to be purchased as part of the primary care trust budget.

Box 1.2 Sex lottery campaign

In 2003, a new £4m public information campaign was launched by the UK government to raise awareness of the risk of STIs among 18–30 year olds. The two-year drive 'Don't play the sex lottery – use a condom' is aimed at young adults on low incomes, highlighted as high risk. A website www.playingsafely.co.uk has been developed to provide information to the target group. The campaign is part of the *National Strategy for Sexual Health and HIV*.[4]

Box 1.3   Health promotion activities

Funded by the public information campaign, the Family Planning Association (FPA) has launched new leaflets on 'Gonorrhoea', 'Genital warts' and
'Genital herpes' in 2003 to add to the first two in the series on 'Chlamydia'
and 'STIs: where to go for advice and help'.

The *National Strategy for Sexual Health and HIV*[4] proposed three levels of
service provision:

- level 1 services to be provided by those working in primary care:
    - sexual history taking and risk assessment
    - contraceptive information and hormonal contraception
    - pregnancy testing and referral
    - cervical cytology screening and referral
    - STI screening for women
    - assessment and referral for men with STIs
    - HIV counselling and testing
    - hepatitis B immunisation
    - targeted screening for chlamydia
- level 2 services to be provided by primary care teams with a special interest
  or by genito-urinary medicine (GUM) clinics or family planning (FP) clinics:
    - long-acting methods of contraception such as intrauterine devices (IUDs)
      or implants
    - testing and treatment of STIs for men and women
    - partner notification
    - vasectomy
- level 3 services to be provided by specialist clinical teams across more than
  one primary care trust:
    - outreach contraceptive services
    - outreach for STI prevention
    - specialist management of STIs including HIV, including coordination of
      partner notification
    - highly specialised contraception and termination of pregnancy services.

The three levels of service provision offer a flexible way of improving the consistency, quality and interprofessional working of delivering sexual health
services. You will notice that there is a greater emphasis on horizontal integra-
tion of different aspects of care so that the services for an individual patient are
not so fragmented. The Strategy also emphasises that all levels of service provision should develop standards of organisation and care.

Information about strategies for sexual health in Scotland is given in the publication *Forum*, a vehicle for exchanging news, views, ideas and information produced by the National Health Service (NHS) Scotland and the Scottish Executive's Directorate of Health Improvement.[7] The expected date of publication of the final document for the sexual health strategy for Scotland is mid-2003. Information about Wales is available in the document *A Strategic Framework for Promoting Sexual Health In Wales*.[8] Northern Ireland remains a special case as there are difficulties in the variations in the legal position there, making it impossible to implement some of the recommendations contained in the sexual strategies for other areas of the UK. For example, the legislation about abortion in Northern Ireland remains unclear as the 1967 Abortion Act does not apply there and many women travel to mainland UK to obtain terminations of pregnancy. Standards for abortion services as described for England would be impossible to set or implement.

At present GUM clinics are in a unique situation. They provide primary care in that patients have open access to their services; that is, patients do not need to obtain a referral from a health professional before attending. They also provide secondary care to those patients who are referred from other health professionals, whether from primary care or from other hospital departments. The medical records that they keep are completely separate from the rest of the patient's medical record kept in primary care or hospital, so that they are held confidentially. Anonymous data about STI rates are collected from these records.

Although all GUM clinics provide diagnosis and treatment for STIs, the other services provided vary greatly. Some clinics provide all contraceptive services, including emergency contraception, others only provide hormonal emergency contraception as part of the treatment for women who have been raped. Some clinics provide advice and treatment for all sexual dysfunctions, including impotence, other clinics always refer elsewhere, and most offer a variable level of expertise. Some clinics provide services for the investigation and treatment of abnormal cervical smears.

What is common to all of them appears to be the increasing number of patients they are being asked to see and manage. Appointment systems have been introduced into many clinics that previously operated a walk-in-and-wait policy. A potential patient has to find the telephone number from a telephone book, a poster in a public toilet or on health premises, or ask someone − not an easy task. For many patients ringing for an appointment can result in their being given an appointment in two or three weeks' time − increasing their anxiety and also the potential for the spread of infection in the interim.

In some areas, amalgamation of FP services with GUM provision has provided a one-stop clinic for patients. In other areas, interchange of health professionals and training of staff in both contraceptive care and GUM have improved the standard of care provided in both services. In larger conurbations, GUM clinics are often the coordinators of outreach services and providers of specialist HIV care and treatment. So GUM clinics may have to provide all three levels of service envisaged in the *National Strategy for Sexual Health and HIV*[4] and, of course, all within present funding and resources!

In order to make the provision of sexual health services comprehensive, we need to think how it can be extended to all who need them. Examples of those poorly served at present include those in prisons and detention centres and those with problems accessing mainstream medical services, such as people with physical disabilities or learning difficulties. Other people also sometimes have difficulties accessing contraception and GUM services. Those who live in country areas may not be able to attend their local general practice during the day because they are working, or attending schools and colleges, and have no access to evening clinics held in urban or city areas because of poor public transport. Even in towns and cities, people working during the day may have problems having time off work – it is difficult to say to your employer that you need time off to go to a GUM clinic – and in many areas, evening clinics are not available. Choice is also a factor to consider. Not all general practices will want to provide all the services at level 1, so services may need to be accessible from several practices. Patients, too, often want to choose what type of sexual health service provision they attend. Evening clinics are more popular than daytime ones, and those staffed by people who are regarded by patients as more approachable, or more knowledgeable, may be preferred. In some areas, asylum-seekers or refugees may have poor provision because of their multiple health needs and the difficulties of finding suitable interpreters. Those from countries with a high prevalence of HIV infection and other STIs may be a great challenge to the general practitioners (GPs) or nurses that they attend.

Primary care

Those working in primary care can expect to have greater involvement in sexual health. We need to set standards for the framework of education and training in the delivery of sexual healthcare. Working through the chapters in this book will help you to achieve them. We also need standards to ensure that services are of consistent quality as well as designing ways of monitoring their delivery. There is an initial inequality to overcome with the addition of services in general practice to those already provided by GUM clinics. Treatment in GUM clinics is free of prescription charges, and provision in general practices or FP clinics at levels 1 and 2 should not disadvantage the users by involving a prescription charge for treatment. The provision of investigative services is also very variable in general practices and FP clinics. In some areas, few laboratory investigations are available, or there are difficulties of transport of specimens to the laboratory. The sexual health expertise of health professionals in general practices and FP clinics also varies enormously.

Developing and increasing the opportunities for networking between GUM and other healthcare providers should improve the quality of sexual health services. At present, referral to GUM services after investigation in a general practice, FP clinic or hospital clinic often leads to patients failing to attend. The referrer is usually unaware that the patient has defaulted from further investigation, treatment or partner notification. Treatment and efforts to prevent spread of infection are occasionally duplicated or, more frequently, not fully implemented. Networking in the future might take the form of shared records or shared staff such as health advisors, as well as joint staff training, secondment or shared posts. The establishment of posts for senior house officers in GUM as part of the training for general practice registrars and the exchange of training between nurses working in FP, practice nursing and in GUM is already occurring in some parts of the UK. Pharmacists play an important role in providing health advice. In most areas of the UK many pharmacists have done extra training so as to play an extended role in providing emergency contraception. Pharmacists give information to customers about obtaining further advice or treatment for contraceptive or STI needs. NHS Direct and, where available, the walk-in NHS clinics, can give information to people about access to suitable sexual health provision.

However, given the level of patient demand for sexual health services in general practices, FP services and GUM clinics, the implementation of the *National Strategy for Sexual Health and HIV*[4] cannot be managed adequately without an investment of additional resources. GUM clinics have been struggling to manage the increase in demand for their services. The increased number of STIs diagnosed, combined with increased demand for testing and treatment which follow publicity campaigns, will put an enormous load onto the existing provision. The principles of rapid and open access must be maintained if the consequences of poor sexual health are to be avoided. Although the actual number of people in the UK infected by HIV is small, the social consequences are potentially large.[9,10] Sexually transmitted infections affect a much larger number of people, causing ill health, relationship problems, infertility, ectopic pregnancy and genital cancers.[11-13] Although unplanned pregnancies do not always result in unwanted children, the large number of abortions carried out each year represents considerable personal distress.[14]

HIV services

Reducing the number of people with undiagnosed HIV infection is another laudable aim of the Strategy. Testing will be offered routinely in GUM clinics and should be made more widely available in other settings as a 'normal' test.

You need to consider the implications of this policy. People offering the test will have to have the knowledge and skills (as well as non-judgemental attitudes) to offer testing and deal confidently with both negative and positive results. If you work in an area with a high level of prevalence of HIV, you need be competent to offer testing. If you work in a rural area with very low levels of infection, you may only need to know where such expertise can be accessed.

At present people with positive results suffer much stigma. Certain groups of people are assumed not to be at risk of HIV (because they are heterosexual or not drug users) and as a result are not offered testing. Wherever you work, you should develop clear standards for what the offer of HIV testing should include, taking account of different settings, different reasons for testing and different population groups. For example, you might explain the risks, benefits, timing and reliability of testing quite differently to a pregnant woman, from the information you give to an intravenous drug user who supports his or her habit with prostitution. Standards are being set out for HIV services and a draft document has been prepared for comments for the Medical Foundation for Sexual Health (a charity supported by the British Medical Association) by an advisory group representing large numbers of stakeholders.[15]

The standards that the Medical Foundation for Sexual Health propose come under a managed service network and include those listed in Box 1.4. If you work in an area where more than a few people are HIV-positive, you will need to think about how general health services are to be provided as well as sexual health services. At the beginning you will be providing testing and care for people with no symptoms, in the interim you will be looking after intercurrent illness, and finally you will be helping with palliative care. All these types of interventions need planning and will increase the demands on primary care services.

Box 1.4 Draft standards for HIV services proposed by the Medical Foundation for Sexual Health[15]

1 *HIV prevention.* All HIV treatment and care will take place within the context of a comprehensive, evidence-based HIV prevention programme integrated with other sexual health promotion initiatives.
2 *Early diagnosis of people with HIV.* The NHS will develop, implement and monitor strategies to encourage the uptake of testing and reduce the number of undiagnosed HIV-infected people.
3 *Empowering people with HIV.* All care will take place within a partnership between people with HIV and care providers so that there is joint decision making and support to adopt and maintain a healthy lifestyle. Services will recognise the impact of HIV infection on an individual and the issues of stigma and social exclusion unique to HIV.
4 *Clinical care of people with HIV.* All people with HIV will have access to comprehensive, specialist HIV treatment and care services and to a

full range of supporting services and medical specialties. All these services will be available irrespective of the site of care.

5 *Primary healthcare for people with HIV.* People with HIV will have access to good quality primary medical and dental care, provided by local networks that are sensitive to the particular needs experienced by those living with HIV.

6 *Social care integrated with healthcare for people with HIV.* All people with HIV will have access to social care services that are responsive, culturally appropriate and tailored to individual need. All people with HIV requiring multi-agency support will receive integrated health and social care.

7 *Sexual healthcare for people with HIV.* All people with HIV will receive comprehensive sexual healthcare integrated with their HIV specialist care.

8 *HIV and pregnancy.* The NHS will develop, implement and monitor policies that seek to empower and support pregnant women with HIV to maximise their health and reduce mother-to-child transmission of HIV.

9 *Care of families with HIV.* Children, their families and carers will have access to specialist adult and paediatric multidisciplinary care, including community care and support.

10 *Emergency care of people with HIV.* All people with HIV will have prompt access to rapid and effective treatment of all emergencies (HIV and others) by appropriately trained clinical healthcare workers.

11 *Care of people with HIV during admission to hospital.* All people with HIV will have access to comprehensive, specialist HIV inpatient treatment and care services and to a full range of supporting services and medical specialties.

12 *Respite, rehabilitation and palliative care services for people with HIV.* All people with HIV will have access to palliative and respite care services that are sensitive to their specific needs at different stages of the disease. Access to rehabilitation services will be dependent on their current needs and potential to improve.

Confidentiality

Concern about confidentiality is the biggest worry preventing young people from attending general practices for help and advice about sexual matters and other health worries.[16] At least walking into a general practice surgery does not label someone immediately as being 'sexually active'. They could be there

---

Box 1.5 Confidentiality dilemma

Tina's mother speaks to the receptionist after collecting her repeat prescription. She says, 'I thought I saw my Tina coming into the surgery while I was parking the car. If Tina's in with the doctor I'll wait for her to come out so I can give her a lift back home.' The receptionist is in a dilemma. Should she say that Tina is here so that she can have a lift home? What if Tina doesn't want her mother to know that she's here or why she is here? She resorts to quoting the rules, 'I'm afraid I'm not allowed to say whether any particular person is in the surgery. Confidentiality, you know.' Tina's mother sniffs in an annoyed way and departs muttering 'Unhelpful receptionists.'

---

for a sore throat or a bad toe and many health professionals recognise the patient who tries out one or two other, often trivial, complaints to try to gauge the reaction of the doctor or nurse before coming to the point of the consultation. Someone attending a sexual health, FP or GUM clinic runs the risk of being recognised upon entering and feeling immediately stigmatised. The more confident people feel about their sexuality, the less embarrassed they feel about seeking out specific sources of help. There is much anecdotal evidence that people do not approach general practices for advice on STIs because of the fear of lack of confidentiality, and that people being tested for HIV in GUM clinics do not want their general practices to be informed of the results. You should ensure that watertight systems are in place to prevent any information about a patient having sexual health needs or risk factors for sexual health problems being released without their consent. Any issues of confidentiality should be clarified before information about individuals is passed to others.

Experienced health professionals and managers may assume that junior or new staff know all about confidentiality, but of course they may not. There are many tricky situations in the workplace where one person may ask for information about another's medical condition (e.g. test results or a progress report) when it is not clear-cut as to whether this information should be supplied or withheld. Even acknowledging to others not immediately involved in the care of that patient that someone is attending or being treated by a service may be a breach of confidence (see Box 1.5).

The Caldicott Committee report describes principles of good practice to safeguard confidentiality when information is being used for non-clinical purposes:[17]

- Justify the purpose.
- Do not use patient-identifiable information unless it is absolutely necessary.

- Use the minimum necessary patient-identifiable information.
- Everyone with access to patient-identifiable information should be aware of their responsibilities.

These principles are useful to keep in mind when dealing with clinical situations as well.

Insurance reports are an example where information is being used for non-clinical purposes and many people do not realise the extent of the information being requested by an insurance company from their GP. Guidelines for completion of insurance reports are available on the website for the British Medical Association (BMA).[18] Their guidelines (salient points are summarised in Box 1.6) point out that the General Medical Council (GMC) states that doctors must:

> Be satisfied that the patient has been told at the earliest opportunity about the purpose of the examination and/or disclosure, the extent of the information to be disclosed and the fact that relevant information cannot be concealed or withheld. You might wish to show the form to the patient before you complete it to ensure the patient understands the scope of the information requested.

These guidelines are kept up to date, so it is in your interest to check them yourself for the most recent recommendations.

Box 1.6   Guidelines for completing insurance reports[18]

- Insurers should not request, and doctors should not reveal, information about an isolated incident of an STI that has no long-term health implications, or even multiple episodes of non-serious STIs again where there are no long-term health implications.
- Other incidents of STIs may have actuarial or underwriting significance and should be revealed with appropriate consent.
- Insurance companies should not ask whether an applicant for insurance has taken an HIV or hepatitis B or C test, had counselling in connection with such a test or received a negative test result. Doctors should not reveal this information when writing reports and insurance companies will not expect this information to be provided. Insurers may ask only whether someone has had a positive test result, or is receiving treatment for HIV/AIDS or hepatitis B or C.
- Doctors are expert in clinical matters and can only give professional advice about those issues upon which they are expert. General medical records hold information about patients' lifestyles, such as smoking, alcohol intake, drug use or sexual behaviour. Only the applicant has accurate information about lifestyle but the insurance industry will use

any information doctors reveal about these matters. Some doctors consider that they should not complete sections of the insurance form asking for this information and will write 'refer to applicant for information' or similar wording. Nevertheless, medical conditions that have arisen as a result of a patient's lifestyle choice are legitimate areas for doctors to comment on with, of course, appropriate consent.

Services for young people

Services for young people should provide an open access service in line with these criteria:

- open to young men and women with an upper age limit of, say, 25 years
- involving young people in planning and evaluation of the service
- with an explicit confidentiality policy highlighting the rights of young people, including those under 16 years, to the same degree of confidentiality as older patients
- staff with non-judgemental attitudes, trained in working with young people
- a non-clinical atmosphere reflecting young people's culture and the diversity of the local community
- a location that offers young people easy access with sufficient anonymity
- opening hours that match young people's availability
- service publicity that is actively disseminated to young people in places where they meet.

A useful publication to consult if you are thinking about setting up or extending services for young people is *Get Real*, available from the Save the Children Fund.[19] This includes information about what is already being provided and more detailed research into five different types of innovations providing targeted sexual health services for young people.

One-stop shops

In the one-stop shop model, the minimum level of service relating to contraceptive and sexual health advice would be extended to include both level 1 and level 2 specialist sexual health services, referred to earlier. Some of the functions at level 3 might also be included, for example abortion or sterilisation services or outreach HIV provision. Many primary care organisations are considering whether this is the preferred way forward to make best use of the limited resources and expertise. In some areas, FP services and GUM clinics have amalgamated to provide joint provision. In other regions, primary care trusts have added the FP services to the provision by general practitioners with a special interest (GPwSIs) to provide extended sexual health services. Elements of these level 2 services include:

- enhanced contraceptive services, including IUD insertion and contraceptive implant insertion
- vasectomy
- testing and treating STIs, including invasive testing for men
- partner notification
- initial investigation and management of infertility
- incontinence
- menopause management
- development, evaluation and monitoring their own services
- providing training and support for other health professionals.

As part of the implementation of the *National Strategy for Sexual Health and HIV*,[4] the Department of Health is asking for volunteer pilot sites to be evaluated until 2006. Consideration will be given to services that do not have all these elements in place but plan to expand to adopt such a model. Pilot sites can be located anywhere across England.

As a minimum, the service must include elements of both STI and contraceptive care and have open access. The service should also undertake a leadership role in terms of sexual healthcare work among local general practices and other local sexual health services. The service is expected to have a data system that allows the routine collection of activity information for evaluation.

The evaluation for the Department of Health by the research team will look at the key issues shown in Box 1.7.

Box 1.7   Key issues for one-stop clinics for sexual health

- The impact of these models on the range of sexual health impact and outcome indicators.
- The impact of these models on actual and perceived service access.
- How these services have developed/are developing care pathways within local sexual health networks which link primary care and specialist sexual healthcare services.
- The acceptability of such services to their target client group.
- The acceptability of such services to service staff, commissioners and staff of other services in the local area.

- The training needed to develop and support these models. This should include the development of enhanced primary care nursing roles in sexual healthcare.
- The expertise and levels of staffing needed to run the services.
- The logistical issues involved with providing care for patients from neighbouring general practices and those not registered, including funding and other resource issues.
- The impact of the service on demand and the impact of any additional workload on the local sexual health network.
- How issues regarding confidentiality and STI regulations are addressed.
- The mechanisms for collecting activity data within the service and the collaborating sexual healthcare network.
- The extent, and success of, the service in building partnerships with agencies outside of health, e.g. youth and social services, education.

If you or your organisation are thinking about setting up, or have already set up, an innovative sexual health service, you may want to look at how many of these measures you can evaluate for your service.

Commissioning sexual health services

The Department of Health has published a toolkit for primary care trusts and local authorities for commissioning sexual health and HIV services.[20] It suggests several ways in which primary care organisations could set up commissioning consortia, headed by a lead commissioner to pool resources across several primary care organisations. They include suggestions on working with voluntary and community organisations to increase the health promotion and community orientated aspects. The document gives details of what should be included at each level of NHS service provision in its Appendix 4. Look at this appendix for the details on what you should be providing at the level at which you work. Appendix 8 of the toolkit gives a useful example of a clinical governance framework and Chapter 3 provides information about how the conclusions from assessing sexual health needs feed into this for the commissioning of services.

References

1 Greenhouse P (1994) A sexual health service under one roof: setting up sexual health services for women. *Journal of Maternal and Child Health* **19**: 228–33.

2 Department of Health (1992) *Health of the Nation. A strategy for health for England.* HMSO, London.

3 World Health Organization (1975) *Education and Treatment in Human Sexuality: the training of health professionals.* Report of WHO Meeting. Technical Report Series No. 572. World Health Organization, Geneva.

4 Department of Health (2001) *National Strategy for Sexual Health and HIV.* Department of Health, London. Also on www.doh.gov.uk/nshs.

5 Ananthaswamy A (2003) Culture shock. *New Scientist* **177** (2379): 42–5.

6 Chambers R, Wakley G and Chambers S (2001) *Tackling Teenage Pregnancy.* Radcliffe Medical Press, Oxford.

7 Williamson J (ed) (2002) *Strategy for Improved Sexual Health.* Scottish Executive Health Department, Edinburgh.

8 Sexual Health Strategy Steering Group (2000) *A Strategic Framework for Promoting Sexual Health in Wales.* Health Promotion Division, National Assembly for Wales, Cardiff.

9 Herdt G and Lindenbaum S (eds) (1992) *The Time of AIDS: social analysis, theory and method.* Sage, Thousand Oaks, CA.

10 Anon. (1988) HIV infection and AIDS in general practice [editorial]. *Journal of Royal College of General Practitioners* **38**: 219–25.

11 Public Health Laboratory Service (2002) Sexually transmitted disease quarterly report: gonorrhoea in England and Wales. *Communicative Diseases Report* **12**: 39.

12 Taylor-Robinson D (1994) Chlamydia trachomatis and sexually transmitted disease. *British Medical Journal* **308**: 150–1.

13 Public Health Laboratory Service (2002) Sexually transmitted diseases quarterly report. *Communicative Diseases Report* **12**: 1.

14 Sonderberg H, Janzon L and Sjoberg NO (1998) Emotional distress following induced abortion: a study of its incidence and determinants among abortees in Malmo, Sweden. *European Journal of Obstetrics* **79**: 173–8.

15 Advisory Group to the Medical Foundation for Sexual Health (2002) *Standards for NHS HIV Services.* BMA, London.

16 Donovan C, Hadley A, Jones M *et al.* (2000) *Confidentiality and Young People Toolkit.* Royal College of General Practitioners and Brook, London.

17 Department of Health (1997) *Report of the Review of Patient-identifiable Information.* The Caldicott Committee Report. Department of Health, London.

18 http://www.bma.org.uk

19 Barna D, McKeown C and Woodhead P (2002) *Get Real: providing dedicated sexual health services for young people.* Save the Children Fund, London.

20 Department of Health (2003) *Effective Commissioning of Sexual Health and HIV Services.* Department of Health, London.

2

How competent are you to provide sexual healthcare and what are your training needs?

We use the term 'competence' here to mean the 'ability to perform the tasks and roles required to the expected standard'.[1] Knowledge and skill are components of competence. Capability is a term that describes 'what a person can think or do'. Whether or not a person's capability makes them competent in a particular job depends on them being able to meet the requirements of that job.[1] Capability implies that individuals can develop sustainable abilities that allow them to adapt to a changing environment and react appropriately to unfamiliar situations.[2]

The standard expected to be able to judge someone as 'competent' will vary with their experience and level of responsibility, and take into account the need to keep up to date with changes in practice. Different people – managers, staff, individuals, patients, clients etc. – will have different expectations of what counts as competence (see Box 2.1).

Box 2.1   What is a competency?

Competency is what you do with what you have got. The underlying personal factors that you have include:

- personality
- skills
- experience
- knowledge
- attitudes
- qualifications.

There can be a gap between competence (what a person can do) and performance (what a person actually does). This gap may be caused by a range of factors – personal matters such as an individual's attitude, personality or mood; environmental factors such as workload, time pressures or working conditions; or situational factors such as a lack of resources or support.

A competency-based approach to training consists of functional analysis of occupational roles, translation of these roles into outcomes and assessment of a person's progress on the basis of their demonstrated performance of these outcomes. The potential advantage of this approach is that training can be flexible. It can be personalised for someone whose current competence is compared against the explicit standards expected for their role and responsibilities and increased public accountability.[3]

It is important to remember that we should anticipate the competencies that individuals will need as service improvements or changes are made, and not just settle for measuring the present state. The competence approach is strengthened when the competence areas identified can be demonstrated in the work setting and are associated with doing the job well.

An example of the competence approach is the Management Charter Initiative (MCI), a description of personal competence for managers. There are four clusters of areas within this – planning, managing others, managing oneself and using intellect. Each cluster is then broken down into dimensions and for each dimension there are a number of behaviour indicators.[4]

Another way of looking at competencies in the health service is to break them down into sectors as below:

1 solving problems
2 meeting the needs of patients and staff
3 achieving personal results
4 being cost-effective
5 using initiative
6 improving performance
7 communicating
8 interacting with others
9 working in teams
10 developing others
11 empowering others
12 keeping focused on the work
13 achieving through others
14 leading others.

Sectors 1–9 apply to everyone; sectors 10–14 apply to those who have responsibility for others. Each sector below has some examples of how you might establish your competency.

1 Solving problems:
- defines the problem to be solved and communicates information to others who need to know
- matches the approach to the complexity or importance of the problem
- decides what information is required to understand the causes of a problem

- analyses the data
- develops options for solving the problem, choosing the one most likely to succeed
- tests the solution
- communicates the solution to those who need to know
- implements the solution.

2 Meeting the needs of patients and staff:
- finds ways of gathering information about the needs of patients and staff
- informs them about things they might want to know
- talks to them frequently
- responds promptly to queries or requests
- asks for feedback on how well their needs have been met
- handles complaints satisfactorily
- actively seeks to improve the ways in which the needs are met.

3 Achieving personal results:
- sets realistic but challenging targets for achievement
- plans and organises own workload
- adopts best policy for efficiency
- controls own progress and use of resources
- maintains commitment in the face of setbacks
- meets agreed targets
- monitors own performance.

4 Being cost-effective:
- seeks best value for money
- works within agreed budgets
- balances standard needed against cost
- thinks about the impact on other people's work or costs
- passes on information about costs to others.

5 Using initiative:
- recognises and acts upon opportunities to do things
- originates activity without having to be asked
- finds ways of removing or reducing hindrances to getting things done
- develops innovative ideas and concepts
- offers ideas in areas where has no direct responsibility
- spots things that fall between people's areas of responsibility and deals with them.

6 Improving performance:
- strives for excellence through continuous review
- seeks and acts on feedback to improve performance
- acts to correct underperformance
- uses new technology and applies new skills
- promotes the positive aspects of change.

7 Communicating:
  - identifies with whom to communicate
  - is precise and clear
  - structures communications logically
  - uses the appropriate medium for communication
  - uses the right style for the communication
  - listens actively and checks understanding before responding.
8 Interacting with others:
  - modifies behaviour by observing the impact on others
  - uses tactics to fit the situation
  - seeks to understand and take account of the other person's perspective
  - challenges others' views constructively
  - uses reasoned argument to support a view
  - accepts challenges to own ideas and responds constructively
  - negotiates agreement that meets both parties' needs
  - builds positive and credible working relationships with others
  - treats other people with respect.
9 Working in teams:
  - shares information
  - asks others for their views and shares own views
  - listens to others' ideas and challenges constructively
  - builds on the ideas of others
  - supports team decisions and puts team needs above personal interests
  - seeks resolution of differences between team members
  - meets commitments given to the team
  - alerts the team when it is deviating from its task.
10 Developing others:
  - helps others to understand the competencies critical to their job and how they can improve
  - identifies individuals' development needs and arranges appropriate development activity
  - helps people fulfil their potential
  - gives constructive feedback
  - acts as a mentor to give personal guidance
  - uses mistakes as a positive opportunity to help learning.
11 Empowering others:
  - manages by involving others and being receptive to ideas and views
  - assesses others' readiness to take responsibility
  - encourages others to make, and take responsibility for, decisions
  - enables others to have responsibility and authority
  - clarifies boundaries
  - helps individuals to build self-confidence

- gives people the freedom to choose how to do things and monitors progress lightly
- arranges for people to acquire the necessary knowledge and skills they need to exploit their personal qualities
- recognises and appreciates people who behave in an empowered way.

12 Keeping focused on the work:
- ensures the aims of the workplace are in accordance with district/regional/national priorities
- sets current work to align with long-term aims
- monitors the need for change
- remains clear about what changes will be needed in the future
- gains support to realise the workplace plans
- identifies, and takes account of, the consequences of actions on other areas
- invests time, effort and money in longer-term planning
- sets current priorities against long-term aims.

13 Achieving through others:
- identifies the workplace plan with which personal plans are aligned
- agrees clear roles and goals with others
- ensures that the individual's plans contribute to the overall plan and priorities
- identifies and drives forward priority targets
- involves others in meeting the targets
- monitors and feeds back progress
- encourages and supports individuals and the team
- fully utilises the team members' skills and attributes.

14 Leading others:
- creates, communicates and secures commitment to a clear objective
- initiates and manages change to progress to the goal
- gives a model of the behaviour expected by the team or organisation
- is visible, approachable and earns respect
- supports own staff especially when difficulties arise
- encourages, motivates and enthuses others
- champions ideas from others that will help to achieve the goal
- provides constructive feedback to the team
- creates a positive climate in which team members can learn and progress.

Think widely about the scope of your work. Training in planning and providing sexual healthcare covers core skills relating to topics such as sexuality and sexual health, as well as issues such as awareness, attitudes, information, communication skills and relationships. Training to develop awareness of cultural differences is also important in understanding and meeting the needs of others who do not share your own current values and understanding.

Providers, advisors and planners must be aware of the difficulties that specific groups face in accessing services and ensure that the services provided meet their needs. Make sure that you and other staff working in sexual health and HIV are properly trained and supported so that all of you can deliver respectful and non-discriminatory care. You should understand and respond to local communities and their cultures by learning from, and supporting, community organisations and individuals. You can help to develop services, in discussion with local service users and organisations, that maximise the take-up from the population groups at most risk. You can build networks with others inside and outside the NHS who serve the target populations.

People need information and services to help them care for themselves. Sexual health services have a core role in providing information on prevention of HIV, STIs and unintended pregnancies. Services like NHS Direct, helplines and NHS walk-in centres also play a part and have a valuable role in improving access to sexual health services.

The *National Strategy for Sexual Health and HIV*[5], or a similar strategy in your region, will dictate some of your training needs, depending on your role and responsibilities at work, and the setting in which you work.

The Audit Commission has studied the current state of education and training in NHS trusts. Recommendations for training and development are stated in Box 2.2.

Box 2.2 Identifying training and development needs[6]

Staff within the NHS should undertake training and development that support their organisation's business plan and the strategic direction of services for patients, while also relating to individuals' and teams' perceptions of need. But many trusts need to improve the identification of training and development needs from business plans, health improvement programmes and clinical governance processes ...

Trusts need to target their resources at providing and commissioning training that is necessary for delivering patient services. They must be able to identify and plan changes in those services. Training needs identified from an individual's point of view are important, but on their own may not reflect longer-term service changes. Trusts should combine bottom-up information identified from individuals with training priorities distilled from business plans, service changes and clinical governance processes. This top-down information also needs to take into account the implications of the health improvement programme and the diversity of the local population.

(Audit Commission)

A training needs analysis will take the form of three stages:[7]

1 identifying the range and extent of training needs from service needs (i.e. expectations in the sexual health strategy and local service delivery strategies)
2 specifying those training needs very precisely. An organisation could do this by pooling the results from the completion by the workforce of the self-assessment questionnaires that follow. Feedback from peers, patients and managers adds other views of the training needs of the individuals
3 analysing how best the training needs might be met.

How to use this self-assessment of your learning needs

You already have basic competency in your present role and for your level of responsibility. You have identified that you need knowledge and skills (and suitable attitudes) in sexual health matters on top of those basic competencies. To help you to find the right level for your needs, first read through the learning needs self-assessment section (Table 2.1) and rate your level in each aspect. Chapters 4–9 in this book are organised for the stage you are at, or want to be, with increasing depth and breadth of knowledge and skills to aid you in acquiring learning. However, this shouldn't stop you reading the sections relating to the other stages as well!

We expect that 'proficient' in our rating scale is roughly equivalent to the expertise required for providing services at level 1 of the *National Sexual Health and HIV Strategy*[5] and the *Implementation* document.[8] If you will be providing services at level 1 of the *National Sexual Health and HIV Strategy*,[5] you should aim to be at least proficient; if you will be providing some services at level 2, you should be aiming at the beginning of the expert level. Then you can build on this by practice and experience and take further training in sexual health to become recognised as expert in your field. As an expert you might be providing services at level 2 or for part or all of level 3, depending on your experience and responsibilities.

The levels of knowledge and skills are graded in the learning needs self-assessment that follows (see Table 2.1) as:

- *Not relevant to post.*
- *Novice.* Knows a little about the sexual health needs of young people and has not generally given advice to young people.
- *Advanced beginner.* Has some knowledge about the subject; is able to direct young people to appropriate services; is able to give a limited amount of advice about the subject.

- *Competent.* Has a good basic knowledge about the sexual health needs of young people and is able to demonstrate this knowledge and skills to others.
- *Proficient.* Has a wide knowledge and is skilled in the subject. Deals with situations presented on a daily basis, advising, treating and managing young people and referring to other agencies when applicable.
- *Expert.* The expert professional has an 'enormous background of experience' and 'intuitive grasp of each situation'. An expert interprets and synthesises information and can handle a wide range of problems in different contexts.[9]

Work through the questions on pages 25–32 to self-assess your current levels of knowledge and skills. This will help you in identifying any specific learning and training needs you may have. You can then set the level that you need to work towards for your particular post or role. It is intended that this book should help you to move from:

- *novice or advanced beginner towards competent (stage 1).* You might be at stage 1 if you have recently started as an additional practice nurse in a general practice that provides drop in services at lunchtimes to young people.
- *competent towards proficient (stage 2).* You might be at stage 2 if you have started working in a FP clinic, in a general practice or in a GUM clinic where services are provided at level 1 and some or all of the services are provided at level 2.
- *proficient towards expert (stage 3).* You might be at stage 3 if you have been working in a service that provides level 2 services and now have to teach other health professionals or make decisions about how services are to be commissioned or provided.

The descriptions of competency in our self-assessment questionnaire were evolved with professionals at workshops, tested out in the field with managers and staff from a wide range of agencies and then revised accordingly.[10] Your self-assessment of the stage you are at should be a global rating of the various components of the aspects described. Our descriptions may seem to cover a wide scope of work tasks and roles, but we have purposely adopted this broad-brush approach. Otherwise we would have become bogged down in the undue detail that would result from breaking down each aspect into minions of small components and arguing over interpretations. Such a narrow approach would be an administrative nightmare and could prove demotivating. We would not propose to reduce someone's job to an exhaustive list of competencies. Look back at the competencies described earlier in this chapter for guidance on what aspects you might wish to consider.

Table 2.1 Self-assessment of your knowledge and skills in respect of sexual healthcare and delivery of services

Please read the statements below relating to sexual health. For each statement circle a number in the box on the right which best describes your level of knowledge for that particular statement.		Stage of your knowledge and/or skills:				
	Not relevant to post	Novice	Advanced beginner	Competent	Proficient	Expert
Example: Aspect 1: Taking a sexual history *'I am aware of the need to reduce embarrassment in others when taking a sexual history, and avoid assumptions about sexual activity, but I still get uncomfortable sometimes. So I would answer 1.'*	0	1	1	2	3	3
Taking and using the sexual history *Aspect 1: Taking a sexual history* Is aware of the opportunities for raising the subject of sexual health in both related and general health encounters. Knows how to reduce embarrassment and deal factually with the information provided. Is conscious of the need to avoid assumptions about sexual activity (that everyone is sexually active, gender of partner, not restarting sexual activity before the postnatal examination, that patient's sexual practices correspond with own, etc).	0	1	1	2	3	3
Aspect 2: Using the sexual history Knows about the relationship between other medical, social and psychological conditions and sexual functioning. Is aware of, and can dispel, common myths and misconceptions about sexual activity and function. Is able to help people come to decisions about their sexual functioning and need for contraception, protection from infection and help with problems.	0	1	1	2	3	3
Contraception *Aspect 1: Access arrangements for contraception and associated services* Knows and can advise about what facilities are available in general and in local area, contact details for helplines, etc. Knows and can advise about what misinformation is commonly believed (e.g. about lack of confidentiality) and can explain why this is untrue.	0	1	1	2	3	3

(continued)

Table 2.1   (*continued*)

Please read the statements below relating to sexual health. For each statement circle a number in the box on the right which best describes your level of knowledge for that particular statement.	Stage of your knowledge and/or skills:					
	Not relevant to post	Novice	Advanced beginner	Competent	Proficient	Expert
Example: Aspect 1: Taking a sexual history *'I am aware of the need to reduce embarrassment in others when taking a sexual history, and avoid assumptions about sexual activity, but I still get uncomfortable sometimes. So I would answer 1.'*	0	1		2		3
Aspect 2: Use of condoms Knows and can advise about use of condoms and what to do if a condom bursts or slips off prematurely. Can demonstrate how to put on a condom. Knows and can advise about any commonly believed misinformation or myths and can explain why these are untrue.	0	1		2		3
Aspect 3: Range of contraceptive methods Knows and can advise about the range of contraceptive methods that are available (oral, IUDs, injection, ovulation prediction methods, barrier methods such as condoms and diaphragms, implants, sterilisation), the advantages and disadvantages of all methods, contraindications, side-effects.	0	1		2		3
Aspect 4: Emergency contraception Knows and can advise about the guidelines for the provision of emergency contraception and the access points for emergency contraception in the local area for various age groups. Knows the guidelines for fitting an IUD as emergency contraception for those under and over 16 years old. Knows and can advise about risk factors for a STI, what screening tests are indicated and what treatment is required if an IUD is fitted. Knows commonly believed misinformation and can explain the accurate facts. Knows what advice pharmacists can give about emergency contraception; what drugs or appliances may be purchased over the counter; what training pharmacists have had in supplying contraception; costs of emergency contraception.	0	1		2		3

Aspect 5: Prescribing of oral and long-acting contraception
Knows and can advise about best practice in prescribing oral or long-acting contraception.

	0	1	2	3

Aspect 6: Sterilisation
Knows about and can advise on male and female sterilisation. Can discuss the advantages and disadvantages of methods. Knows about any associated short-term and long-term health risks. Can discuss the myths and misinformation about these methods.

	0	1	2	3

Sexually transmitted infections

Aspect 1: Background of STIs
Knows and can advise about the different kinds of STIs that occur in the UK; how common they are locally and nationally; how the prevalence might vary in different groups of people.

	0	1	2	3

Aspect 2: Risks of people catching STIs
Knows and can advise about grading sexual activity into high-, medium- and low-grade risks. Knows and can advise about any commonly believed misinformation or myths associated with sexual health (e.g. catching diseases from a toilet seat) and can explain why they are untrue.

	0	1	2	3

Aspect 3: Contact tracing of STIs
Knows and can advise about the importance of contact tracing STIs, why it is needed, how and where tracing takes place and by whom – both in general and locally. Knows and can advise about the exact procedure. Knows and can negotiate about the options for contact tracing with an infected person when they are partially cooperative or uncooperative.

	0	1	2	3

(continued)

Table 2.1 (continued)

Please read the statements below relating to sexual health. For each statement circle a number in the box on the right which best describes your level of knowledge for that particular statement.	Not relevant to post	Stage of your knowledge and/or skills:			
		Novice	Advanced beginner	Competent	Proficient	Expert

	Not relevant to post	Novice	Advanced beginner	Competent	Proficient	Expert
Example: Aspect 1: Taking a sexual history '*I am aware of the need to reduce embarrassment in others when taking a sexual history, and avoid assumptions about sexual activity, but I still get uncomfortable sometimes. So I would answer 1.*'	0	1	1	2	3	3
Aspect 4: Identification and treatment for STIs Knows and can advise about the evidence for what types of treatment are best practice for treating the range of STIs for men and pregnant and non-pregnant women. Knows how, where and when to refer people for treatment who may or definitely have STIs. Knows and can advise about whether treatment can be bought from pharmacies or needs a prescription. Knows and can advise about preventing recurrence and whether follow-up treatment is needed. Knows and can advise about barriers to treatment – personal and organisational.	0	1	1	2	3	3
Pregnancy *Aspect 1: Pregnancy* Knows and can advise about where people can obtain a pregnancy test; when a pregnancy test is needed. Knows and can advise about the reliability of tests and timing. Knows and can advise about the methods of referral for medical or other help when pregnancy is confirmed. Knows what the conception rates are both nationally and locally for all age groups, including under-16 year olds; variations with socio-economic background or other personal characteristics; variations in age of male partner, outcome of pregnancy (e.g. likelihood of termination); legal issues, ability to give consent.	0	1	1	2	3	3

Aspect 2: Teenage parents
Knows and can advise about education, work opportunities, housing qualification and support systems available in a local area for teen mothers; statistics for employment and career opportunities. Knows and can advise about how a teenage mother may access the practical, social, educational, financial and other support and to what they are entitled.

0 1 1 2 3 3

Sexual violence
Aspect 1: Childhood sexual abuse
Knows and can advise about what situations may be classified as sexual abuse in males and females. Is able to relate to people who have experienced sexual abuse and provide professional help. Knows how and can act – practically and legally. Knows and can advise about establishing systems to check that those who work with young people do not have a history of abusing others. Knows and can advise about what personal support or support services are available locally and nationally to those who have experienced sexual abuse or are in fear of it and the service contact details. Knows and can advise about how long support is likely to last, and what forms it might take. Knows and can advise about any misinformation and is able to explain why this is untrue.

0 1 1 2 3 3

Aspect 2: Sexual violence in adults
Knows and can advise about what constitutes definitions of rape and 'date' rape in heterosexual and homosexual cases; the factors making rape more likely. Is able and knows to whom to refer an alleged rape victim and the support systems in place to deal with this. Knows and can advise about what examination the victim will require in order to give accurate information to the police. Understands how the person who has been raped feels and is able to demonstrate empathy with them. Knows and can advise about the personal and health risks taken by prostitutes and how these can be minimised. Understands and can advise about the difference between willing prostitution and coercion.

0 1 1 2 3 3

(continued)

Table 2.1 (*continued*)

Please read the statements below relating to sexual health. For each statement circle a number in the box on the right which best describes your level of knowledge for that particular statement.

	Not relevant to post	Stage of your knowledge and/or skills:				
		Novice	Advanced beginner	Competent	Proficient	Expert

Example: Aspect 1: Taking a sexual history
'I am aware of the need to reduce embarrassment in others when taking a sexual history, and avoid assumptions about sexual activity, but I still get uncomfortable sometimes. So I would answer 1.'

	0	1	1	2	3	3

Relationships

Aspect 1: Sexual relationships among young people
Knows and can advise about the age young people start to have sex. Understands and can advise about what constitutes social norms for the usual age of first sexual intercourse, types of sexual activity, peer pressure to have sex, numbers of partners. Knows about and is able to advise young people about problems with relationships.

	0	1	1	2	3	3

Aspect 2: Practical support available to people for building relationships
Knows and can advise about local support offered to people of varying ages in respect of interpersonal relationships. Knows how to and when to refer young people to such organisations. Knows how to, and is able to teach or show people how to, build worthwhile relationships.

	0	1	1	2	3	3

Confidentiality

Aspect 1: Confidentiality within all statutory and voluntary services available to people
Knows and can advise about the confidentiality that people of all ages, including young people under 16 years, can expect from a GP, surgery staff, FP clinics, teachers, hospital staff and all other allied services.

	0	1	1	2	3	3

Aspect 2: Rules of confidentiality
Knows and can advise about what a code of confidentiality should contain and how to implement such a code; knows how and is able to monitor that confidentiality is sustained. Knows what to do if confidentiality is breached and can act. Knows and can advise in what circumstances confidentiality can be broken in the interests of a person. Knows how confidentiality is explained to new members of staff.

	0	1	1	2	3	3

Self-esteem

Aspect 1: Understanding of importance of self-esteem
Knows how and can gauge level of self-esteem in other people; knows the association between low self-esteem relating to early pregnancy and risk taking in young people. Knows scales or methods of assessment of self-esteem.

	0	1	1	2	3	3

Aspect 2: Raising self-esteem
Knows and can advise about methods that can be employed to raise self-esteem and self-confidence in people from various socio-economic backgrounds and ethnic cultures.

	0	1	1	2	3	3

Cultural and religious attitudes to sex and sexual health

Aspect 1: Knowledge of sexual health services
Has specific knowledge and can advise about the availability of local sexual health services for people from ethnic minorities or various religions; the barriers that obstruct people from different cultures and religions from accessing services or types of contraception.

	0	1	1	2	3	3

Aspect 2: Cultural differences in relation to sexual behaviour and sexuality
Knows and can advise about cultural differences in attitudes to under-age sex, and sex before marriage for people from various backgrounds, cultures and religions. Knows and is able to explain any cultural and religious differences in expected norm sexual behaviour. Able to advise people from different ethnic or religious backgrounds about sexual behaviour, sexual health, contraception.

	0	1	1	2	3	3

(continued)

Table 2.1 (*continued*)

		Stage of your knowledge and/or skills:				
Please read the statements below relating to sexual health. For each statement circle a number in the box on the right which best describes your level of knowledge for that particular statement.	Not relevant to post	Novice	Advanced beginner	Competent	Proficient	Expert
Example: Aspect 1: Taking a sexual history *'I am aware of the need to reduce embarrassment in others when taking a sexual history, and avoid assumptions about sexual activity, but I still get uncomfortable sometimes. So I would answer 1.'*	0	1	1	2	3	3
Aspect 3: Variations in cultural attitudes relating to abortion and contraception Knows and can advise about how various ethnic cultures and religions perceive abortion and contraception; the frequency of abortion and use of contraception in different cultures and religions; barriers and drivers to abortion and contraception in various cultures.	0	1	1	2	3	3
Screening and investigations *Aspect 1: Cervical smear screening* Knows and can explain to patients the local guidelines for eligibility for cervical smear screening. Can counsel patients about the advantages and disadvantages of screening for cervical cancer. Is aware of the misunderstandings that occur about screening and can discuss these with patients. Understands the results and can explain these to patients. Knows how to obtain further investigations and/or treatment.	0	1	1	2	3	3
Aspect 2: Other screening Understands the principles behind other screening procedures, why some have been introduced and others have not, and can explain the reasons to others. Can discuss the advisability and disadvantages of screening for chlamydia, breast cancer, risks of thrombosis and prostate cancer.	0	1	1	2	3	3

Matching the stages you are at in your self-assessment with learning from this book

The various sections of Chapters 4 to 10 that follow are marked in the right-hand margin to give you some indication of what someone might be expected to know or do in each area of knowledge or skills for stages 1, 2 and 3. Match these stages to the information you have gathered from the self-assessment exercise (Table 2.1) about the stage you are at for each area and the stage at which you are expected to work in your current post or a future role in respect of:

- taking and using the sexual history (Chapter 4)
- screening and investigations (Chapter 5)
- contraception, including emergency contraception (Chapter 6)
- STIs (Chapter 7)
- men's health (Chapter 8)
- pregnancy (Chapter 9)
- sexual violence (Chapter 10).

Other relevant areas are covered within the book and integrated into the text throughout these seven chapters. Look out for the icons shown below:

confidentiality =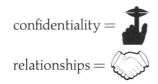

relationships =

cultural and religious attitudes to sex and sexual health =

self-esteem =

If you are new to thinking about sexual health matters so that you are mainly at a novice level across your self-assessment of your training needs, you may want to start reading from the beginning of the book and continue to the end. You will come across a lot of what you need at your stage on the way.

Alternatively, you might prefer to dip in and out of the book, finding the level of information for the stage at which you rated yourself in your self-assessment. To some extent people will perceive the stages at different levels if they are working in very different work environments. What may appear to be at stage 1 if you are working in a specialised service may seem to belong at stage 3 if you are working in the community with young people and their general needs. So find the stage at which you, personally, will be learning to match your own learning needs.

You could use the book to check that the information here is the same as what you thought you knew in your everyday work. If it isn't, you had better use some of the further reading or the references to find out which is right!

Making self-assessment of your training and learning needs more objective

The disadvantage of self-assessment is that it is liable to be excessively subjective. It is difficult to compare the level of self-assessments by different people as some will tend to be harsh on themselves, whilst others will be over-generous in gauging the extent of their knowledge and skills. Your assessment may change as you learn more and become more aware of what you do not know. You may have become arrogant about your ability because others rarely challenge it, either because you work in isolation or because of your seniority or attitudes.

You can increase the objectivity of your self-assessment by involving other people in the exercise to give you feedback on your performance. This might be your line manager at a performance review or a colleague with whom you work. You might complete the self-assessment exercise in relation to your current role and responsibilities, or linked to a job you expect to do in the near future to anticipate what knowledge and skills you will need to acquire.

Alternatively, you might supplement your self-assessment by gathering evidence of your knowledge, skills or performance by other mainly objective methods[11] such as:

- structured peer observation of your knowledge and skills at work
- audit methods
- significant event audit
- risk assessment
- monitoring access and availability, systems and procedures
- feedback from patients or clients
- comparing your management of a case or aspects of your performance with externally set standards.

Learning styles

Now you are clear what you need to learn – what do you do next?

Everyone has their preferred learning style(s) and yours will dictate how you wish to learn what you now find you need to know. Honey and Mumford have described four learning styles:[12]

1 *Activists* like to be fully involved in new experiences, open-minded, will try anything once, thrive on the challenge of new experiences but soon get bored and want to go on to the next challenge. If this is you, you will learn best through new experiences, short activities, and you will want to have a go at things or brainstorm ideas. You might want to take a post in a new working environment, e.g. in a GUM clinic if you work in general practice or family planning, to give you the stimulus to learn.

2 *Reflectors* like to stand back, think about things thoroughly and collect a lot of information before coming to a conclusion. They are cautious, take a back seat in meetings and discussions, adopt a low profile, and appear tolerant and unruffled. If this is you, you will learn best from situations where you are allowed to watch and think about activities before acting. You may like to observe others at their work on an attachment and discuss what you have seen and learnt with a mentor or tutor afterwards.

3 *Theorists* like to adapt and integrate observations into logical maps and models, using step-by-step processes. They tend to be perfectionists, detached, analytical and objective. They reject anything that is subjective, flippant and lateral thinking in nature. If this is you, you will learn best from activities where there are plans and models to describe what is going on. You will enjoy reading books, listening to lectures and attending structured workshops.

4 *Pragmatists* like to try out ideas, theories and techniques to see if they work in practice. They will act quickly and confidently on ideas that attract them and are impatient with ruminating and open-ended discussions. They are down-to-earth people who like solving problems and making practical decisions, responding to problems as a challenge. If this is you, you will learn best when there is an obvious link between the subject and your job. You may wish to learn by constructing a protocol for your workplace or team.

Think about how to structure your learning. If you have to work by yourself, how can you remain motivated and check that you are assimilating the learning? If you can, join in with others as you will find learning more enjoyable and stimulating.

Learning resources

Resources that you might use are given in the Appendix together with a list of relevant websites and organisations.

References

1 Eraut M and du Boulay B (2000) *Developing the Attributes of Medical Professional Judgement and Competence.* University of Sussex, Sussex. Reproduced at http://www.cogs.susx.ac.uk/users/bend/doh.

2 Fraser SW and Greenhalgh T (2001) Coping with complexity: educating for capability. *British Medical Journal* **323**: 799–802.

3 Leung WC (2002) Competency-based medical training: review. *British Medical Journal* **325**: 693–6.

4 Management Charter Initiative (1992) *Middle Management Standards.* Pocket Directory. MCI, London.

5 Department of Health (2001) *National Strategy for Sexual Health and HIV.* Department of Health, London. Also on www.doh.gov.uk/nshs.

6 Audit Commission (2001) *Hidden Talents: education, training and development for healthcare staff in NHS trusts.* Audit Commission, London.

7 Bee F and Bee R (1997) *Training Needs Analysis and Evaluation.* Institute of Personnel and Development, London.

8 Department of Health (2002) *The National Strategy for Sexual Health and HIV. Implementation.* Department of Health, London. Also on www.doh.gov.uk/nshs.

9 Benner P (1984) *Novice to Expert.* Addison Wesley, London.

10 Milson G and Chambers R (2002) *Competence of Professionals and Others Who Work with Young People, in Relation to Sexual Health.* Centre for Health Policy and Practice, Staffordshire University, Stafford.

11 Wakley G, Chambers R and Field S (2000) *Continuing Professional Development in Primary Care: making it happen.* Radcliffe Medical Press, Oxford.

12 Honey P and Mumford A (1986) *Using your Learning Styles.* Peter Honey, Maidenhead.

3

Sexual health needs assessment: an example of a user involvement model

The *National Strategy for Sexual Health and HIV*[1] expects that commissioning sexual health services to meet patients' needs will reduce the transmission of sexually transmitted infections and unintended pregnancies. Each health authority in England should have carried out a sexual health needs assessment to identify the gaps (or any unnecessary overlaps) in local service provision by April 2003.

This chapter describes an example of a sexual health needs assessment and reports the issues, problems and solutions experienced. The fieldwork of this sexual health needs assessment was carried out in South Staffordshire by a team from Staffordshire University and focused on young people in the locality.[2] The model developed can be adapted to assess the sexual health needs of the general population or of any particular group using sexual health services.

What is a health needs assessment?

The *Sexual Health and HIV Commissioning Toolkit for Primary Care Trusts and Local Authorities*[3] identifies needs assessment as the variable foundation of a framework for the future development of sexual health and HIV services. That is to say, needs assessment is essential for commissioners to identify the strengths and weaknesses in service provision within their locality, providing an opportunity to tailor future service provision to the needs of the local population. The Toolkit[3] goes on to describe the linked process from the needs assessment to the delivery of health outcomes (see Figure 3.1).

The key processes are cyclical, where their outcomes will ultimately provide information for the continuing assessment of need. They can be used to find new ways of working so that the local population health needs are met.

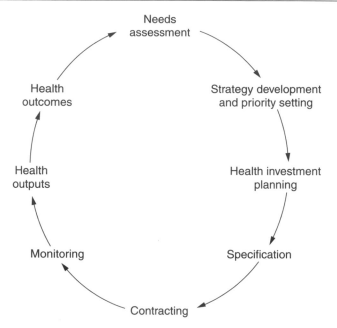

Figure 3.1   The linked process.

A health needs assessment has three components:

1 a description of the health problems of a population
2 identifying inequalities in health and access to services
3 determining priorities for the most effective use of resources.

Put simply, a health needs assessment is a balance of what should be done, with what can be done and what can be afforded.[4]

Identifying whose needs require assessing

The health problems of the population being studied (number 1 above) require a definition of the population being studied. In an assessment of sexual health needs, it is the people who require assistance with their sexual health either in preventive or curative services. The Toolkit highlights the importance of user involvement throughout the commissioning process, by contending that user involvement should not be a token involvement but 'a thread running through the commissioning process'.[3] Effective commissioning demands partnership working between commissioners, service providers and service users. However, there are barriers to user involvement in sexual health and HIV services, such as the stigma associated with accessing such services and the level of confidentiality required within the services. These barriers could be overcome by utilising a number of different mechanisms for service user and community involvement, such as:

- patient advice and liaison services (PALS)
- patient forums
- local authority scrutiny
- commission for patient and public involvement in health.[3]

So in practice when identifying the health needs of your local population, define what you want to do and the component tasks. These might be to assess the sexual health needs within a locality with the objective of improving local services and addressing inequalities (number 2 above). This in turn should reduce the transmission of STIs and the number of unwanted conceptions (meeting number 3 above). Identify the vulnerable groups who are most likely to indulge in risk-taking behaviour. Concentrate on assessing their needs. For instance, in our example in this chapter, the sexual health of young people (12–24 years) is of particular concern,[5,6] making their sexual health needs a priority which should be considered separately from those of other population groups (meeting number 3 by determining priorities for the effective use of resources).

Identifying the barriers

It is very tempting for service providers to blame lack of funding or resources as an excuse not to deliver a service that meets the needs of its service users. We should use existing resources to the best possible advantage. By identifying the barriers to people accessing the services, policy makers and service providers may be able to tailor existing services to meet the needs of users. Identify barriers by asking questions such as:

- *Lack of knowledge of consequences of risk-taking behaviour.* Are those who need to, accessing the service? If not, why not? Is it because they are unaware of their need to access a service? For example, in the case of a sexual health needs assessment, if individuals are not aware of the risks of their sexual behaviour, they will not attempt to access a service.
- *Lack of knowledge of local services.* Is it because they are unaware these sexual health services exist? Are there insufficient public advertisements of the services? Is it difficult for potential users to identify what services are available?
- *Inaccessible services.* Is it because people are unable to access the service because they are unable to travel to it or it is not open when they are able to go? Are they unable to obtain access because of waiting times for appointments or because delays in answering the telephone deter them?

- *Lack of characteristics perceived by the service users as essential for an ideal service.* If people have had a negative experience, or know others who have had bad experiences, they will not usually access the service in the future. Being made to feel unwelcome, having to wait excessively or not having your needs met all make you not want to attend again.

Define what the health problem is

To assess the sexual health needs of young people requires definitions of the terms 'sexual health' and 'health needs assessment'. Goldsmith's definition of sexual health incorporates three essential components:[7]

- sexual expression and enjoyment without exploitation, oppression or abuse
- absence and avoidance of sexually transmitted diseases and disorders which affect reproduction
- control of fertility and avoidance of unwanted pregnancy.

A health needs assessment includes measuring the extent of the problem and assessing the effectiveness of the interventions. A health need is the ability to benefit from a healthcare intervention. However, as a health need should incorporate environmental and social needs, then any health needs assessment should include community participation, equity and multi-agency collaboration.[8]

Pulling the team together

Project manager

Appoint a project manager to organise and ensure that the process detailed within the model is followed. An individual who is familiar with the particular health needs that are being assessed is an advantage. The project manager should not be too entrenched in one particular aspect of the service as this could introduce an unrealised bias to the assessment process. The project manager should be answerable to a strategic steering group.

Strategic steering group

This should be made up of a partnership of local service commissioners and service providers, as ultimately they will be responsible for determining priorities within the existing resources. This strategic steering group should not be confused with the service users' steering group.

Service users' steering group

This group will be directing the approach to the needs assessment itself and should be made up of a group of potential service users who live in the geographical area. It should ideally represent the groups most at risk from the health hazard being assessed (unprotected sex in this example), together with a range of relevant professionals (see Box 3.1).

Box 3.1

In the sexual health needs assessment undertaken in South Staffordshire, the steering group was made up of four young people aged between 15 and 17 years old, the project manager and assistant project manager.

Project assistants

It is essential to consider the whole geographical area covered by the sexual health needs assessment. This ensures that all the barriers faced by potential service users are identified as they may differ from area to area. For example, the solutions required may be different in an urban area to those of a rural area. The geographical area being assessed might be divided according to established working boundaries. A project assistant from each of these areas might be employed to carry out a mapping exercise of local services and to run focus groups and interviews involving service users and potential service users in the area. The project assistants' local knowledge will be useful for working with local professionals working in the field and young people so that the whole of the geographical area is represented (see Box 3.2).

Box 3.2

In the sexual health needs assessment undertaken in South Staffordshire, the geographical area was divided into the localities of the five primary care trusts.

Making the initial plan

The first task is the development of a strategy and/or protocol setting out the purpose and aims of the sexual health needs assessment along with a clear plan of how the aims are to be achieved (see Box 3.3).

Box 3.3

In the sexual health needs assessment in our South Staffordshire example, the purpose was to: 'identify the extent and possible gaps in sexual health services for young people in South Staffordshire, by undertaking an assessment of the sexual health needs of young people aged 12 to 24 years old, across South Staffordshire'.[2]

Consider the scope of the assessment by identifying:

- who is most at risk and whose needs should be assessed
- who are the professionals or individuals being contacted on a regular basis.

For sexual health, national reports[3,5] identify those most at risk from unwanted conceptions and STIs as including young offenders, young people leaving care and young parents. These young people come into contact with teachers, probation officers, social workers, midwives, voluntary workers, school nurses, youth workers and police officers etc. on a regular basis. It is important not to limit your assessment to those professionals and individuals already providing or receiving sexual health services. You must also identify those individuals who are not accessing services to discover what barriers there are to people accessing existing services.

Collecting data: qualitative stage

Stage 1: development of focus group schedules

Focus groups help to elicit views about services. Members of the steering group and the project manager should compile focus group schedules: one for the focus groups of professionals and another for the young people's focus groups. The schedules will stimulate discussion and keep the participants to the task. This is especially valuable when discussing topics that are normally considered to be socially taboo, such as sexual matters. Each focus group from the various geographical areas must use the same schedule (see Box 3.4).

Box 3.4

The schedules used in the focus groups of the South Staffordshire sexual health needs assessment are in the Final Report.[2] You can reproduce or adapt them.

Stage 2: arrange focus groups of professionals

Organise focus groups of professionals and others working in the field in each of the geographical areas. The project assistants should recruit a whole spectrum of participants from the professionals and others from across the geographical areas being assessed (see Box 3.5).

Box 3.5

In the South Staffordshire health needs assessment, professionals and individuals who worked with, or had a responsibility for, young people were invited. These included teachers — in general and those who taught sex and relationships education — as well as youth workers, social workers, school nurses, police officers, project workers, youth offending teams, pharmacists, general practitioners, FP nurses, genito-urinary medicine nurses, midwives, practice nurses, police officers, voluntary sector workers, individuals working with young offenders and those leaving care, others working with young people who had been sexually abused and professionals working with young parents, young carers, homeless and black and ethnic minority young people.

Each focus group consisted of up to 12 individuals from the list above and each discipline was represented over the five focus groups of professionals. The professionals were each paid £20 for attending.

Representatives from professional organisations (such as Connexions — see Appendix), which have been recently set up, should be considered for inclusion in future assessments of young people's needs. Other groups such as foster parents and those working with young gays and bisexuals would also be valuable additions to future assessments.

Stage 3: arrange focus groups of young people

The project assistants might recruit up to 12 people as potential service users from each of the geographical areas. Ideally, the people attending the focus groups should be representative of both high-risk and geographical groups of people (see Box 3.6).

Box 3.6

In the South Staffordshire sexual health needs assessment we held a focus group of young people in each of the five geographical areas. We concentrated on the potential service users being representative of the geographical area rather than trying to identify people being at risk from their sexual behaviour. The young people were each paid £5 vouchers (phone or book) for attending.

Stage 4: develop an interview schedule

Interviewing individuals from the professionals' and service users' groups allows you to gain more in-depth information than is likely to emerge from the focus groups. By including this stage, you will be able to explore some of the ideas and experiences that emerge from the focus groups (see Box 3.7).

Box 3.7

In the South Staffordshire sexual health needs assessment, we gained a more detailed picture of the current sexual health services by interviewing two individuals from the steering group, and from the professionals' and potential users' focus groups. The interview schedules were derived from the qualitative data gained in the focus groups by members of the steering group and the project manager.[2]

Stage 5: one-to-one interviews with professionals

The project assistant could conduct one-to-one interviews with volunteers or selected participants from each of the focus groups. Try to ensure that the professionals that you interview are not from the same or similar professions, so that they represent a cross-section of the professionals working in the field.

Stage 6: one-to-one interviews with service users and potential service users

The project assistant could conduct one-to-one interviews with volunteers or selected subjects from the focus groups. Try to ensure that the interviewees reflect varying population groups experiencing differing health risks, so that they represent a cross-section of potential service users.

Collecting data: the quantitative stage

Stage 1: develop measures of health need and desired service characteristics

Use the qualitative data you have collected to develop a measure of potential service users' needs and identify the barriers to their needs being met. Members of the steering group and the project manager should work on evolving the measure together (see Box 3.8).

Box 3.8

In the South Staffordshire sexual health needs assessment we developed a measure in the form of a questionnaire. The questionnaire was divided into several sections. The first identified the knowledge of young people about the consequences of risk-taking behaviour. (We established this first because if young people did not have this knowledge they would not realise their risk and would therefore not even try to access sexual health services.) The second section dealt with their knowledge and perceptions of existing services and from which sources they got their knowledge. The third section attempted to discover what the characteristics of an ideal sexual health service are for young people, from the point of view of the respondents. Finally the questionnaire asked when and where they would like sexual health services to be sited.

Stage 2: distribute the measure

The measure can be distributed to a sample from each of the high-risk groups of potential service users across the geographical areas being assessed (see Box 3.9).

Box 3.9

In the South Staffordshire sexual health needs assessment, we distributed 2000 questionnaires to a representative sample of young people drawn from each of the five geographical areas. Around 1300 questionnaires were returned, mostly by post or by the representatives of the organisations who distributed them. For example, the midwives who had young parents as their clients would distribute the questionnaire and envelopes. Completed questionnaires were returned sealed and the midwives would send them back. Some organisations had freepost envelopes for individuals to return their responses themselves.

Stage 3: analysis of data

The data can then be analysed either manually or, better still, by a data analysis computer package to hone down on population subgroups by locality or type of risk group.

Write your final report

Write up the results in the form of a report discussing the issues identified by the assessment and containing recommendations for service providers and policy makers to use when planning future service provision (see Box 3.10).

Box 3.10

In the South Staffordshire sexual health needs assessment, a number of main themes have been identified from the data examined so far:

1 *A dichotomy between what professionals and young people want from service provision.* Overall the quantitative data revealed a dichotomy between

what professionals and the young people wanted from service provision. Professionals emphasised health promotion, i.e. educating young people as to the consequences of risk-taking behaviour and providing health promotion material (i.e. action before the act). The young people stressed 'damage limitation', such as action after unprotected sex had occurred, access to emergency contraception or treatment of STIs (i.e. action after the act).

2 *Professionals' lack of knowledge of services.* There was a general lack of knowledge of local services by the professionals, with most assuming sexual health services meant contraception services. However, there were exceptions within the groups with some respondents having a good knowledge base. There was a particular lack of knowledge of GUM clinics with one professional asking: 'What is GU anyway?' One professional stated: 'How can we expect young people to know about services when we do not know ourselves?' Many professionals highlighted problems in disseminating information to the 'grass roots' and would welcome the opportunity to be able to network with other professionals on a regular basis.

3 *Young people's lack of knowledge of services.* Young people's knowledge of services was as poor as the professionals'. Young people seemed to be aware of FP clinics but unsure about what happens there. They also highlighted the inadequacies of the services they did know about. Among the responses from the South Staffordshire young people's focus groups to 'What sexual services are available in your area?' were:

> 'Just the family planning clinic. We can get free contraception from the clinic. It runs on a Monday. I think it should be open more. It's only open on a Monday evening, 7–10 p.m.'
> 'What if you need emergency contraception?'
> 'They should have it in pub toilets.'
> 'You can't get emergency contraception in pub toilets.'

4 *Lack of services for young people under the age of 16 years.* Some GPs are willing to see under-16 year olds without an adult present to give them sexual health advice. Some will see patients for contraception services who are not registered with their practice for general services. Others are not comfortable about seeing under-16 year olds without an adult present. General practices are not allowed to advertise what they do, so information about their services is passed on through word of mouth. Some agencies like Emerge (a support group for those who have been sexually abused) are not allowed to have under-16 year olds referred to them.

5 *Lack of services for young males.* Young men generally felt that FP clinics were predominantly a female service. They were perceived as being

staffed by female nurses (and usually are). Young people preferred a gender-specific service, in that young women wanted to be seen by a female and young men by a male health professional.

6 *Confidentiality, anonymity and privacy of services were the greatest concerns for young people.* To meet these concerns the most common proposal was for drop-in centres where advice and information were available on a number of different issues, not just on sexual health. The staffing of these centres is an important consideration as not only do they have to have the skills necessary to provide the relevant advice, but also the ability to communicate with young people. One young 14-year-old male stated that he would most like to see 'someone who didn't ask loads of personal questions'. This was consistently the most predominant factor in what young people felt was the most important characteristic of an ideal sexual health service. One young female explained how she felt when accessing a sexual health service: 'It's really embarrassing. You don't want your Mum to know. You don't want someone saying "I've just seen your daughter getting condoms free".' It was generally agreed by young people that they would prefer a general service specifically for young people, one that had open access and was available after school and at weekends.

7 *Particular barriers for people from black and ethnic minority groups.* The confidentiality and anonymity barriers were reported to be particularly acute for young people from black and ethnic minority groups. According to cultural expectations, most of these young people are not expected to visit their GP on their own. The GP is acceptable to them as someone able to give sexual health information. Professionals emphasised the importance of consulting with religious and community leaders to obtain support, with one professional saying: 'We need culturally appropriate services for young people.'[2]

As indicated previously, a health needs assessment involves these three parts:

1 A description of the health problems of a population.
2 Identifying inequalities in health and access to services.
3 Determining priorities for the most effective use of resources.

The final report of the assessment should contain a description of the health problems of the local population (part 1) and the recommendations should identify the inequalities in health and access to services (part 2). The final stage of the needs assessment is for the strategic steering group to utilise the assessment findings and determine the priorities for the most effective use of resources (part 3) (see Box 3.11)

Box 3.11

In South Staffordshire the results of the interim report were used to set up and deliver a multi-agency training course for professionals and those who work with, or who have a responsibility for, young people in the county. This was aimed at professionals being enabled to deliver sexual health information and advice to young people. These training courses provide individual professionals with an opportunity to network with others who work with young people. Information packs are provided which contain information on all local services, contact numbers, appointment times and access arrangements. The information packs also contain information on how to obtain health promotion materials such as leaflets and posters. Early evaluations show that these courses are increasing professionals' confidence in supporting young people and being able to direct them to the most appropriate services.

How this model informs commissioning of sexual health services

In the *Sexual Health and HIV Commissioning Toolkit for Primary Care Trusts and Local Authorities,*[3] Appendix 8 gives an example of a clinical governance framework for professionals providing sexual health services. This framework is based on a primary care clinical governance model. You might like to look at other models of clinical governance in the publication *Making Clinical Governance Work for You.*[9]

Examining this model more closely you can see where the sexual health needs assessment fits in. It underlies all of the provision of health services, for, without knowing what is needed, you cannot begin to evaluate what progress you are making towards meeting those needs. It is no good providing all sorts of services that no one wants, needs or is going to use! On the other hand, you might not provide services that are badly needed or not provide enough of them. So although all the parts of the following framework are important, none can exist without establishing what needs they are meeting.

Clinical governance framework modified from the Toolkit[3]

Quality assurance measures to maintain standards are suggested for *all* of the quadrants described below and include:

- confidentiality
- appropriateness
- availability
- continuity
- coordination
- safety
- respect and caring
- timeliness.

First quadrant

Health professionals and their employers will need to ensure that they are able to provide a range of clinical services or tasks outlined in this quadrant. The tasks described are for a 'generic' professional providing a sexual health service, the balance of which will depend on the nature of the service and the health needs of the clients seen — that is, determined by the sexual health needs assessment.

You can alter the tasks to show individual aspects of professional activity in more detail. Clearly, appropriate training and qualifications are essential. Primary care organisations and their employees have a dual responsibility to ensure that they are appropriately qualified to undertake the tasks expected of them and to remain up to date. Quality assurance in professional activity should develop a needs-led, evidence-based and consistent approach. This is largely the responsibility of individual health professionals and teams. If shortfalls are identified these should be made known to the primary care organisation managers. This quadrant is within the primary care organisation and includes:

- history taking, examination, diagnosis and treatment
- diagnostic tests, including for pregnancy
- referral to other agencies
- screening tests
- counselling
- prescribing and dispensing
- undertaking procedures/operations
- follow-up and ongoing support
- partner notification
- team approach
- health promotion
- provision of training
- keeping patient records and data collection
- participation in continuous professional development
- undertaking audit and research.

Second quadrant

This identifies in broad terms the important links that health professionals need in order to undertake their clinical work. These links, that are external to primary care, need to be recognised, promoted, developed and fostered by primary care organisations. Many of these organisations or individuals will have been identified in the sexual health needs assessment as already providing services or in need of development in some way. They include links between primary care and:

- maternity and gynaecology services
- pathology and radiology services
- general medicine, paediatrics and dermatology
- GPs, health visitors, school nurses, dentists, pharmacists, dietitians and other professionals allied to medicine
- youth and community services
- child protection services
- social services
- schools and colleges
- drug agencies and HIV services
- Brook and other voluntary organisations
- Benefits Agency
- police
- public health
- health promotion.

Third quadrant

This section lists the organisational support that health professionals require when undertaking their clinical work. Responsibility to ensure adequate provision of this essential non-clinical support lies with the primary care organisation. A comment by each entry shows how the sexual health needs assessment might inform these support services. You might think of some more examples from your own or other people's experiences:

- clerical and administrative support – enough staff to answer the telephone promptly and well enough trained to answer queries clearly
- information technology (IT) systems – to make appointments easily, keep records confidential and yet accessible when needed, provide look-up facilities when staff do not have an answer to hand and help to monitor standards

- site location and facilities appropriate to tasks – provide welcoming and easily accessible premises open at convenient times
- appropriate equipment and supplies, and storage space – to be able to provide the clinical service required at the time
- appropriate caseload/workload – the staff are not too busy to sit down and listen to what people need
- efficient patient record systems – to be able to record patient information once, accurately and reliably, and make it available when it is required
- pathology collection systems – so that tests can be done in a timely way and as accurately as possible
- sterilised supplies/sterilisation procedures – so that procedures can be done safely
- published service standards that are monitored – to demonstrate that standards are being reached
- security at workplace – so that patients and staff are safe and do not feel threatened
- recruitment and retention policies for appropriately qualified staff – people know what they are doing and can give good service
- robust recruitment arrangements for those working with young people – with the right attitudes and checked for safety
- human resources and employment policies supportive of part-time and multisite working – staff who know what real life is like
- financial support and time to enable personal and professional development etc. – staff who have time to keep healthy and up to date
- user consultation and robust complaints procedures – to try to prevent things going wrong and put things right if they do
- service promotion and advertising – so that users know what is available, when and where.

Fourth quadrant

This section contains community and district health needs underlying the sexual health service and is directly informed by the sexual health needs assessment. Some of the national and local policy contexts in which sexual health services are operating are also included. Both health professionals and primary care trusts should be aware of the content of this section, although it is mainly derived from outside of the primary care setting:

- community profiles/health needs assessment
- local delivery plans (LDPs) and the local teenage pregnancy strategy
- government strategies, e.g. teenage pregnancy, sexual health and HIV[1,5]

- Fraser (Gillick) guidelines
- venereal disease regulations and other public health law[10]
- Abortion Act[10]
- child protection procedures[10]
- government publications such as *Organisation with a Memory*, Data Protection Acts 1984 and 1998, Caldicott guidelines, Access to Medical Records Act, Crown guidelines on nurse prescribing[9]
- Nursing and Midwifery Council (NMC) and GMC guidance
- advice from the Medical and Nursing Royal Colleges and English Nursing Board
- National Institute for Clinical Excellence (NICE)
- health and safety regulations[10]
- Medicines Control Agency guidelines
- national voluntary organisations.

This clinical governance framework demonstrates clearly that a sexual health needs assessment underpins all of the commissioning activities for sexual health services and that primary care trusts need to seek the widest professional advice and support from those involved in the provision of services.

References

1 Department of Health (2001) *National Strategy for Sexual Health and HIV*. Department of Health, London. Also on www.doh.gov.uk/nshs.

2 Cunnion M and Ryan K (2003) *Sexual Health Needs Assessment of Young People in South Staffordshire – Final Report*. Staffordshire University, Stafford.

3 Department of Health (2003) *Effective Commissioning of Sexual Health and HIV Services: a sexual health and HIV commissioning toolkit for primary care trusts and local authorities*. Department of Health, London.

4 Wright J (1998) *Health Needs Assessment in Practice*. BMJ Books, London.

5 Social Exclusion Unit (1999) *Teenage Pregnancy*. The Stationery Office, London.

6 Public Health Laboratory Service (2000) *Trends in Sexually Transmitted Infections in the United Kingdom, 1990–1999*. Public Health Laboratory Service, London.

7 Goldsmith M (1992) Family planning and reproductive health issues. In: H Curtis (ed) *Promoting Sexual Health: proceedings of the Second International Workshop on Prevention of Sexual Transmission of HIV and Other Sexually Transmitted Diseases*. Cambridge 24–27 March 1991. British Medical Association Foundation for AIDS, London.

8 World Health Organization (1986) *Ottawa Charter for Health Promotion: an international conference on health promotion*. WHO, Geneva.

9 Chambers R and Wakley G (2000) *Making Clinical Governance Work for You*. Radcliffe Medical Press, Oxford.

10 Beresford N and Branthwaite M (2003) *Law for Doctors*. Royal Society of Medicine Press Ltd., London.

4

Taking a sexual history and what to do with it

In Chapters 4–10, look out for the numbers and icons (see page 33) in the right-hand margin that indicate the learning stage (1, 2 or 3) and other relevant areas.

Why do you need to take a sexual history?

The health professional is usually the person first contacted when patients have **1** problems with their sexuality or with a sexually transmitted disease. It is important that the health professional discovers the reason for the consultation otherwise the problem may not be resolved, and this may be harmful to patients and their sexual partners. Patients often present their problems in disguise because of fear that they will be criticised or condemned if they are honest about the real reason for their attendance.

You cannot help a person decide on the best method of contraception for themselves unless you understand something about their sexual life, plans for the future and lifestyle.

Most health professionals have had little training in taking a sexual history, diagnosing STIs or helping patients with simple sexual problems. Health professionals often suggest methods of contraception that they think would be best for the patient, rather than exploring and then listening to what the patient might prefer. Discomfort with the areas of sexuality can discourage practitioners from approaching the subject or discussing it with patients.

Sex has become a common topic of discussion in the media and is mentioned **2** more often in social conversation in the UK. There is more openness about sexual problems and about STIs. Fear of AIDS, knowledge about herpes or chlamydia, expectations of a rewarding sexual life – all bring patients in for advice and help. Patients are more willing to bring their sexual health problems to health professionals nowadays than they were in past years and they expect to obtain professional expertise.

Increasingly as well, proactive preventive medical health promotion is expected of health professionals, rather than just reactive illness care. Sexuality and its problems are more likely to be encountered when screening for cervical cancer, giving contraceptive advice or when mammography or testicular self-examination are being discussed. The challenges that health professionals have barely started to tackle include the prevention of common infections like chlamydia, the prevention of pelvic inflammatory disease in young women and the detection of STIs that so often give no symptoms.

Reasons for discomfort when starting to talk about sex may include:

- fear of offending the patient
- unfamiliarity with the patient's culture (ethnicity, sexual orientation)
- unwillingness to become involved in complex and time-consuming issues.

If the healthcare provider does *not* ask directly about sexuality, the patient is unlikely to volunteer the information on their own. Studies indicate that healthcare providers know less than half of the patient's sexual concerns.[1] Even when directly asked, someone may be reluctant to talk about their sexual life because of:

- embarrassment about their sexuality
- worries about confidentiality
- the presence of a partner
- concerns about being judged inadequate or odd.

Despite the importance of sexual history taking, fewer than 15% of new patient visits include an adequate sexual history. Patients often do not specifically discuss sexual concerns unless prompted by the clinician, but a failure to mention sexual matters does not mean they have no sexual concerns.[1] The health professional may be reluctant to raise the issue of sexual concerns as well, but has a responsibility to do so.[2]

By following some simple guidelines to increase the patient's comfort level, most primary care providers can become skilled at obtaining a sexual history and making appropriate decisions about diagnosis and treatment or referral to other clinicians with specialised training. Most health professionals start by using a standard protocol that increases their own comfort level, but soon learn what is most relevant for an individual patient. They can tailor the gathering of information by paying attention to the feedback from the individual about what is most important.

An anonymous postal general health survey in four general practices showed that 44% of men and 36% of women reported that they had sexual dysfunctions (of various types) and that 23% of men and 15% of women would like help for their problems.[3] The GP was the person most of them wanted to approach, with women being more likely to want help from someone of the same gender. The next best choice of help for women was the FP clinic, and for men, the GUM clinic. So patients believe that primary care is the right place to ask for help with their sexuality.

What is 'normal sexual activity' in Western culture?[4,5]

The median age of first intercourse in the UK is 17 years for both men and women. Looking at findings from surveys of those who are currently teenagers, 20% of women and 28% of men started having intercourse before the age of 16 years. That means, contrary to what many teenagers (and adults) believe, that 80% of young women under the age of 16 years are *not* having sexual intercourse. The young people who do start sexual intercourse early are most at risk of unplanned pregnancy as nearly half the women and over half the men under 16 years did not use contraception at the time of first intercourse.

1/2

About 75% of the population regard premarital sex as acceptable, but nearly 80% say that after marriage, sex outside marriage is unacceptable. However, a study in 1985 showed that 66% of males and 30% of females had had extra-marital affairs, perhaps more a case of 'do as I say not as I do'.[4] Extramarital affairs certainly cause much upset, anguish, marital breakdown and expense.

Most surveys suggest that couples who live together have sex about one to two times a week — more often in the first year and showing a gradual decline with age. It can vary a lot, and many couples are happy with more or less.

In 1943, a study suggested that most heterosexual encounters took less than two minutes, but over the years information about love-making for pleasure has increased the time and satisfaction for many couples.[4]

Masturbation is common: 99% of men and 66% of women report that they have masturbated.

Seventy-five per cent of men and 70% of women report experience of oral sex at some time.

Anal sex is not legal in the UK and often regarded as immoral. It is likely to be under-reported, but 14% of men and 13% of women say they have experienced anal intercourse in heterosexual encounters.

Regarding homosexual practice, about 6% of men report genital contact of some type with other men and about 3% of women with other women at some time in their lives.

You might want to look at some, or all, of the reports on sexual attitudes in Britain[4-8] and compare the most recent survey reported in 2000 with the previous one carried on in 1990. The reports give you considerable information about sexual activity and how this affects sexual health.

3

General reminders about taking a history

Taking a history from patients about their sexual life and activity should follow **2**
the same rules as for taking any medical history:

- Make sure you are ready for the patient, then welcome them, ensuring their
  comfort and privacy. Know and use the patient's name and introduce and
  identify yourself. Guard against making assumptions from the appearance of
  patients, but notice the impact that their appearance has on you.
- Use open-ended questions initially. Negotiate a list of all issues, but avoid
  detail at this stage. Note any specific requests (e.g. for a repeat of medication). Clarify the patient's expectations for this visit. You may need to ask
  the patient 'Why have you come about this now?'
- Elicit the patient's story.
- Return to open-ended questions directed at the major problem(s). Encourage
  the patient to talk with silence, non-verbal cues and verbal cues. Focus on
  the problem by paraphrasing and summarising.
- To make the transition from their account to your agenda, summarise the
  interview up to that point and say something like 'I'd like to ask you a few
  questions so we're clear what to do.'
- If it is necessary to use an interpreter, select one who has experience in medical interpretation and understands the importance of confidentiality. Before
  using an interpreter of the opposite gender, consider the impact on the
  patient's openness in responding to questions. Using a partner or a child as an
  interpreter will create even greater constraints.

How can you take a sexual history?

- Explain the reason for taking a sexual history. This reduces the possibility **1**
  that the patient will be offended or misinterpret your intentions. Ask the
  patient if it is all right to carry on.
- Tell patients about confidentiality – mention this early on and explain how
  the information they give you will be kept confidential and who will have
  access to that information.
- Listen carefully – allow patients to guide the discussion and introduce the
  terminology. This does not imply that you should use the same language or
  slang as they do. Most patients will tell you most of what you need to know
  (and what they want from the consultation) in the first three minutes if you
  do not interrupt them.

- If the patient agrees, consider asking their partner to participate. However, also allow for one-to-one discussion. This is especially important as some issues involve sexual activity with other partners or information that one of a couple would not want the other to hear.

A check-list of questions on sexual activity

Nurses or doctors need to know some information to make sure that the advice, investigations or treatment are based on the fullest history within the time constraints of the consultation. There is a lot of information that you might need to obtain.

A list of possible questions is given below – but you will not need to ask all of these! When you first start to take a sexual history you might want to have a check-list and ask the questions from this list that apply in that particular consultation. Obviously you would not ask a man about periods or a young woman about menopausal symptoms, or a young man or any woman about prostate symptoms. Guard against making assumptions – anyone who has sexual intercourse may be at risk of STIs, whatever their status, culture or appearance.

Be careful about the words that you and the patient use. The vagina or uterus mean something specific to you, but the terms may be used in a much wider sense by patients to indicate any part of the female genitals. Similarly, someone may talk about 'going to bed with someone' and you need to be clear whether this actually includes sexual penetration. 'Making love' may include sexual penetration, or may refer to caressing and other sexual stimulation. There are problems too with identifying the sex of the partner – 'Pat' or 'Lesley' could be either. Always check that what you understand is what the patient meant.

Keep in mind at all times the main reason why the individual came to see you. Don't ask something just because it is in a check-list or in case it might be useful later – the person will just get irritated and think you are wasting time on your agenda instead of focusing on theirs.

Most of these questions apply equally to men and women. You will not include all of them with every individual, but you may find it helpful to check that you have not missed out something important after listening to the patient. If you have, think about whether this is because it is difficult for the patient to talk about (and they have avoided the subject) or whether it really was not relevant. You may find that other things come up as you progress through the consultation. Keep in mind the main reason for the patient's attendance – you may want to leave some information to one side at this stage.

- Are you currently sexually active?
- Do you have any worries about your sex life?
- Do you have more than one sexual partner?
- Do you have sex with men, women or both?
- Tell me about your sexual activity. For example, do you have oral sex? (Other forms of sexual activity should also be specified, depending on the patient's sexual orientation. This is particularly important if you need to investigate for a STI. For example, you will need to know the areas of the body that might become infected – throat, rectum etc. – so that investigations are complete but relevant.)
- What about masturbation?
- Are you sexually satisfied?
- Is your sexual activity as frequent as you would like it to be, or is it too much or too little?
- Does your partner prefer more or less sexual activity than you do?
- Do you have orgasms?
- Do you have pain with sexual activity?
- Does your partner(s) have pain with sexual activity?
- Is there anything that you would change about your sexual activity?
- Have you any worries about your genitals?

Menstrual and obstetric history (women only)

- At what age did you begin menstruating?
- When was your last menstrual period?
- Have you ever had unprotected intercourse? If so, when and how often?
- How long do/did your periods last? Are/were they regular? How often do/did they occur?
- Do/did you ever experience bleeding, pain or discomfort during your period or during intercourse?
- Do you have any problems with premenstrual syndrome?
- Are you experiencing any menopausal symptoms such as . . . ? (Give examples like hot sweats.)
- Have you ever had pregnancy-related problems? (Give examples like raised blood pressure.)

2

Pregnancy intentions (both men and women)

- Do you plan to have a child?
- If so, how soon would you like to become a parent?

- Do you need any advice on getting pregnant or on care during pregnancy?
- Have you any worries about your fertility?
- If you do not want to become a parent at present, are you and your partner protecting yourselves from pregnancy? If so, how?

STIs (both men and women)

- Have you ever had a STI?
- Do you think you are at risk of getting a STI?
- How many sexual partners have you had in the past 12 months?
- Have you ever experienced burning when you pass water?
- Have you had any discharge from the penis or soreness of the genital area?
- Have you had any rash or lumps in the genital area?

Prostate health (men only)

- Have you felt the urge to urinate frequently or had dribbling when you urinate (pass water)?
- How many times do you have to get up to pass urine at night?
- Have you noticed any reduction in the flow of urine?
- Do you have any lower abdominal pain?
- Do you have pain on ejaculation?

Hepatitis (both men and women)

- Have you had yellowing skin or eyes (jaundice), or have friends told you that you look yellow?
- Have you had upper abdominal pain, light-coloured stools or dark urine?
- Have you ever been told you had a liver problem/hepatitis?
- Have you been vaccinated for hepatitis?

Alcohol and drug use (both men and women)

- How many alcoholic drinks do you have each day? Beer, wine or spirits?
- Is alcohol or drug use interfering with your life?
- Does your use concern you or your friends and family?
- Have you ever got in to trouble because of drug or alcohol use?

Medication use (both men and women)

- What prescription medications are you currently taking?
- What over-the-counter, non-prescription medications are you taking?
- Are you taking herbs, vitamins or supplements? If so, which ones?

Physical, sexual and emotional abuse (both men and women)

- When you were young, did anyone ever touch you in a way that made you feel uncomfortable?
- When you were young, did anyone ever ask you to, or make you, touch their body in a sexual way?
- Has anyone ever hit or battered you?
- Do you live with anyone who verbally abuses you?
- Have you ever been forced to have sex against your will?

Medical or surgical trauma (both men and women)

- Have you had any injuries to your genitals or any surgery on your genital area?
- Have you had a vasectomy?
- Have you had a hysterectomy or sterilisation?
- If you have had children, were the deliveries normal?
- Have you been treated with chemotherapy or radiation therapy?
- Have you any worries about your genitals?

Selective information gathering   3

With more experience you will not need to use a check-list. Many of the questions above will not be relevant anyway and you will be able to spend more time discussing what the individual came to deal with. Particular areas may need special attention depending on what answers you obtain. For example, you may want to give someone time to talk about an abusive relationship, especially if it is the first time that they have been able to mention it. If someone becomes distressed about something in their past history – e.g. a termination of pregnancy, an operation or treatment for infection – you will want to explore why this is upsetting for them. The distress may be due to misunderstandings that can be corrected, or the person may just need an opportunity to talk about something that cannot be discussed with others.

Risks of STIs, including HIV

Never assume that because a patient is older, they are not at risk for STIs. Older adults embarking on new relationships after separation, divorce or death of a long-term partner may be at particular risk. After the 16–26 year age group, the next peaks in rates of STIs and HIV are among those aged 45 years and older. Questioning about a history of STIs should specify the various types, e.g. gonorrhoea, chlamydia, warts, HIV, syphilis. If an answer is affirmative, follow-up questions about treatment of both the patient and partners are essential.

Menstrual and obstetric history

Women may be reluctant to bring up symptoms associated with the peri-menopause or menopause, but it is clearly important to be aware of these symptoms in order to provide good healthcare. Pregnancy-related problems, such as injuries from forceps and vacuum extractions, can result in chronic pelvic pain, painful intercourse and urinary or faecal incontinence.

Atrophic vaginal and vulval soreness and dryness after the menopause, or sometimes when breast-feeding, can cause sexual difficulties that may be just accepted by the patient as 'normal' or something she cannot ask about.

Pregnancy plans

Given the current trend in developed countries to delay child-bearing and the increasing number of pregnancies among women over 40 years of age, it is important to discuss pregnancy issues with this group. Many women may not realise that the possibility of pregnancy remains real even after menstrual cycles become erratic and that protection from unintended pregnancy is important until they are truly menopausal. This is usually stated as one year after periods have stopped if the woman is over 50 years, or two years without periods if she is younger, although evidence for this is based on experience.

Alcohol and drug use

Both can lead to sexual dysfunction. Some people may substitute the 'high' of drug use for the pleasure of sexual activity and alcohol can be a potent cause of depression. Lack of funds for the purchase of alcohol or illegal drugs can lead to prostitution. Prescribed drugs may have unwanted effects on sexual function.

Medications

Both prescription and over-the-counter medications may affect sexual functioning. Women may not consider hormonal therapy as medication, so it is important to specify it as an example. Similarly, herbal nutritional supplements may have oestrogenic-like effects or be problematic in their impact on sexuality.

Physical, sexual or emotional abuse

Avoid asking bald questions about 'abuse' but offer people the opportunity to express their opinions about episodes that they found upsetting or disturbing.

Don't assume that only women are abused; always include history of sexual abuse and rape when taking a sexual history from both male and female patients. Use open-ended questions such as 'Did anyone ever do anything to you when you were younger that made you feel uncomfortable or distressed?'

Medical or surgical trauma

A broad range of medical and surgical treatments can adversely affect sexual function. Often people undergo treatments that affect their sexuality without advance knowledge or understanding that this is a likely outcome. Conversely, there may be mistaken impressions about the effects of surgery such as hysterectomy or prostate operation. Case studies have been reported in which a patient, her partner or both assumed that the vagina was removed as part of hysterectomy. Men may believe that they will be unable to achieve an erection after a prostate operation. Both the patient and partner need to be informed about how any surgery or treatment such as chemotherapy may affect sexuality.

When can you take a sexual history?

You may need to explain to a patient why you need to know about their sexual history. It may not be obvious to the patient why you are inviting information on sexuality, if it is not in response to an overt presentation of a sexual problem. For example, 'Some people find that going on to treatment for blood pressure affects their sexual life. Have you noticed any difference since you started on this treatment?'

You might enquire whether sexual intercourse is satisfactory after a hyster-ectomy, a prostate operation or after a myocardial infarct, or whether the short-ness of breath with respiratory diseases such as asthma or chronic obstructive airways disease causes problems with intercourse. Ask people with arthritis or back pain how they manage their sexual activity.

Asking children and young people

You will not normally need to enquire about sexual matters with children **2** unless there is an obvious reason.

The older the child, the more appropriate it becomes to take a sexual history. To omit taking a sexual history from a teenager with cystitis, vulval or penile soreness, or a genital rash might be negligent. Young men may be worried about discharge from the penis as not all of them are aware of the normality of 'wet dreams'. Similarly, young women may be concerned about the changes in vaginal secretions throughout the monthly cycle, especially if they think no discharge should be present.

If a child has a vaginal discharge or perianal warts there may be child **3** protection or legal considerations. You may need to think about referral at an early stage. Explaining that you do not have the necessary skills to sort out the problem that needs investigation is just as routine in this case as it would be for any other field in which you do not have expertise.

Adults and sexual history

Most adults are not offended if you ask if they are sexually active as part of a **2** general enquiry. As we become older our perception of who is sexually active changes. Teenagers cannot believe that anyone more than 10 years older than themselves can still be sexually active, but the older we become the more we become certain that sexuality continues into old age. Most pensioners are pleased to be asked, although their activities may be restricted through lack of available partners or infirmity.

Although contraceptive and infection problems are less common as people **3** get older, sexual difficulties and dysfunctions increase. Many people can be helped to look at alternative ways of managing their sexual activity from the ways that worked well when they were younger. They may need to look at alternative positions, more stimulation, making sexual activity last longer or taking pain relief or anti-anginal medication beforehand.

Gender and sexual history

Women attend primary care more often than men. It is often easier to obtain a **2**
sexual history because they attend for contraception, pregnancies and intimate
examinations such as cervical smears.

Men between 16 and 50 years of age attend primary care infrequently and
often only for urgent conditions such as accidents and infections. You would
not talk about sexual health promotion at such consultations (unless clearly
related to their sexual lives such as a STI), but they can be invited to attend for
a well-person check.

Well-person checks, the registration medical for new patients or a consultation for travel immunisations may provide the perfect opportunities for dealing
with sexual health promotion, enquiries about contraception or sexual health
problems. It is relatively simple to add sexual health screening questions to a
general medical history taken in the context of a well-person check. In women,
information often flows naturally from questions about contraception, pregnancies or gynaecological conditions. In men, complaints about urination or
bowel disorders can provide a useful start.

You may want to introduce the subject by asking if the person lives alone or
with a partner and then move on to the particular (as you do with other
systematic enquiries). You might ask if they have any problems with their sex
life, if the contraceptive method used (if any) is satisfactory and if there has
been any change in partner recently.

Physical disability

The media projects images of sexual activity being for the young and attractive. **2**
People with physical disabilities have the same rights to fulfilling and safe
sexuality as everyone else. They may have special difficulties with sexual activity. Sex education, information, family planning and advice are less accessible to
people with disabilities. Audiotape or Braille information leaflets are even less
common than those available in minority languages. Access to surgery premises
or clinics is frequently difficult. Carers are protective and often treat the people
with disabilities as children with no sexual needs or desires. It is sometimes
difficult for health professionals to consult privately with someone with a
disability – the carer brings them into the room and stays to assist, preventing
private conversation. Think how you could consult privately with a patient in a
wheelchair in your consulting room or clinic, at the patient's home or in a residential or nursing home.

People with learning difficulties

Some of the difficulties listed above may also apply. It is often difficult to talk without the carer being present, who often answers for the patient. The carer may be more embarrassed than either the patient or the health professional and prefer to deny that sexuality is the problem. Development of interest in sexual activity for the first time at an older age can lull the carer into a false sense of security – growing adolescent-like interest in sexual activity at the age of 26 years can be quite a shock. Health professionals may find themselves dealing with the confusion of the carer as well as the patient's problem. Problems with lack of knowledge, slowness of comprehension and idiosyncratic names for parts of the body are hurdles in the path of clear discussion of sexual health. Use pictures, models or even dolls to demonstrate what you are discussing, break each communication into shorter parts and check after each section to ensure that both you and the patient understand.

Psychosocial problems

Anxiety, depression and relationship problems are often associated with sexual difficulties. Health professionals are aware that sexual desire will be lowered in depression. Most also know that anxiety may cause loss or inhibition of erection and loss of vaginal lubrication in women. Similarly, sexual incompatibility or inadequacy may cause or be associated with insomnia, emotional distress or partnership disputes.

Asking how the partner feels about the emotional problem, or enquiring directly whether the condition has affected sexual feelings and activity, is frequently helpful in establishing the extent, and sometimes the causes, of the current problem.

Contraceptive consultations

Most people do not want to use contraception. Their priority is to be able to have sexual relationships. In order for a couple to use contraceptives, the perceived disadvantages of using a method of contraception have to be overcome by the need to avoid pregnancy. The wish to avoid a sexually transmitted disease is even less of a priority for most couples. Decisions about sexual relationships are usually made in private, but to obtain most methods of contraception a health professional has to be involved. The more difficult it is to consult that health professional, the less likely someone is to do so. Organising the delivery of contraceptive care is an important part of enabling people to choose, use and continue to use contraception.

Interviews for contraceptive advice need to concentrate on the needs of the patients. You should be helping patients to understand how their sexual behaviour and the choice of contraception affects the risk of STIs as well as pregnancy. Looking at the implications of sexual behaviour is very important in choosing and in using a suitable method to prevent both risks. You may want to encourage using a condom for prevention of infection *in addition* to providing a good method of preventing pregnancy.

Sometimes people will want a really effective method, for example when starting a new relationship, new job or when learning a new skill. At other times, it would not be such a disaster if they did become pregnant and a less effective method may become more acceptable. Similarly, as women become older their fertility declines and less effective methods become more reliable; however, they may want an even more certain method if a pregnancy would seriously disrupt their lifestyle or ambitions!

How well am I doing?

Think about checking your history-taking ability. We all like to think that we do it really well, but most of us can improve if we look at what and how we are doing. You could use video recording and review your skills with a trusted colleague. Ask your colleagues for feedback if they are seeing the same patients (did you deal with their concerns, did they remember what you said, did they understand you?). You could use patient satisfaction questionnaires, look at significant events or complaints or preferably, use all of them from time to time.[9]

Sexual problems

Whether you welcome it or not, patients will ask for your help with their sexual problems. Most problems can be managed within the normal working consultation of health professionals. Embarrassment or a lack of common language for sexual parts or practices may cause extra difficulties. Never assume that you know what the problem is, or what has caused it. Be an active, thinking listener and establish clearly what the problem is for each individual. If the information you have is insufficient, think *why* you have not been told about particular aspects of the problem. It is not enough just to ask lots of questions, but also to understand why you might need to ask them.

Patients can present openly with problems of lack of desire, performance or satisfaction. They may test you out before revealing the real reason for their consultation. Covert presentations are common. The sexual difficulty may be hidden because the patient is not aware of the connection between it and the problem presented (e.g. pain, soreness or dislike of contraception). Sometimes, the sexual difficulty is hidden because of fear of ridicule, disapproval or of the consequences of revealing it.

Investigate only when indicated by the history of the complaint. Undertake screening investigations if there is a clear benefit, such as checking the blood sugar and blood pressure in a man with gradual onset of impotence.

Refer as part of a joint decision. Understand that some patients find it difficult to consult a familiar health professional with sexual problems. You may find the problem too complex, or too distressing, to manage yourself. You cannot refer appropriately before you understand the nature of the problem.

Often, explaining the problem to a professional with good consulting skills can enable patients to understand the problem or find a suitable solution for themselves.

Sexual history and sexual difficulties

Most people will be able to tell you what the problem is and, by looking at it with you, discover what is the right thing for *them* to do to put it right. By the end of the patient's account you will usually know:

2

- when the problem started (i.e. is the problem primary or secondary)
- if anything happened at the time it started (could this be causally related or is it misleading?)
- if it always happens or if it is connected to any particular circumstance or person (this may help with identifying difficult personal relationships or environments)
- why the person has presented now (pressure from a partner, a trigger from changed circumstances etc.).

If you have not identified any of these factors, think about *why* you have not.

There may be defences put up by the patient because they do not want to tell you. A woman may not tell you that she had exciting orgasmic sex with a previous partner if she is afraid that her present partner will discover that she compares him unfavourably. You may not be told about something that happened at the time the problem started because it seems too trivial to mention. For example, until the doctor drew out the timing of the event, one patient had not made the connection between her resentment and loss of libido with her husband who had thought she made too much fuss when her cat was run over.

The event may seem too terrible (to the patient) to be told. One woman was convinced that she had to control her sexual feelings (and lost her desire for sex with her husband) because she had felt excitement when she witnessed a stripper at a cricket match. She was appalled at what she regarded as a totally inappropriate and shocking response.

Be an active thinking listener, not a passive receptacle for information. Pay attention to what is going on between you and the patient. For example, do you feel protective, bored or irritated with the patient? Does it throw any light on how that patient relates to others outside the room?

You may find that you hear more problems about people's sexuality as you become more confident at allowing patients to set their own agenda for what they tell you. You might want to do some more reading[10,11] and perhaps attend some further training (see websites in the Appendix for further information).

3

Dealing with sexual problems

Sexual difficulties are common but can present as a hidden problem. Patients expect doctors and nurses to ask about sexual functioning, but many health professionals have had little education and training about sexuality. Personal attitudes may inhibit skills and influence patient management. Key features in the history are whether the problem is primary or secondary, what else happened around the time the difficulty began, and whether it happens consistently or only in certain circumstances. The way patients react in the consultation with the doctor or nurse may shed light on the manner in which they relate to significant others in their sexual life.

1

Physical examination is an important tool. It not only establishes the physical findings, but, if carefully observed, can also reveal as much non-verbal material as the history. Investigations are rarely needed and should be guided by the history, not ordered routinely. Treat each person as an individual with a unique problem and do not assume that this problem for this patient has the same cause or solution as was true for the last person you saw for this complaint. Always keep in mind fears that people have about the confidentiality of what they may tell you. This may have implications when you offer a chaperone for any physical examination, as discussion of your findings may need to be postponed until you cannot be overheard.

Sexual problems are common in the general population. The prevalence varies according to how people are asked and the definition of what represents a

2

problem. Dunn's questionnaire survey of 4000 randomly selected patients in four general practices found that the prevalence of one or more defined sexual dysfunctions was 44% in men and 36% in women.[12] This large cross-sectional study indicated that sexual problems cluster with self-reported physical problems in men and with psychological and social problems in women. This implies that effective help for sexual problems could have a broad impact on health in the adult population.

Health professionals need to approach the topic with therapeutic attitudes, in order not to communicate their own anxieties to the patient. Most health professionals learn about sexuality from reading and experience. Without specific education and training, they are often unaware how much their own background, upbringing and prejudices influence what they learn and how they respond to patients. Guidelines from professional organisations emphasise the importance of not allowing personal views about a patient's lifestyle, sexuality or age to affect the treatment that health professionals give.

You might look back to the guidelines on taking a sexual history (p. 58) to remind yourself of the importance of taking a sexual history in a competent and sensitive way.

Criticisms have been made that the pharmaceutical industry has been creating a **3** new 'illness' of sexual dysfunction in order to profit from marketing 'cures'. Most people will not need pharmaceutical intervention and can be helped by being given an opportunity to discuss their sexual lives in a non-judgemental way. Others may be helped to regain confidence in managing their sexual lives by judicious introduction of pharmaceutical assistance. Expectations of perfect performance (whatever that is) are fuelled by media portrayals of unreal situations and the lack of openness in (British) society prevents a more realistic perspective.

Physical examination in sexual problems

Patients bring their problems to a health professional because they perceive **1** that the problem may be physical as well as, or instead of, psychological or social. A physical examination accepted or welcomed by the patient can be very helpful. You may find a physical reason for the problem, or the absence of a finding (such as pain) can help the patient to face the possibility of a psychological or social cause.

For a physical genital examination, offer a chaperone or offer to postpone the **2** examination until one is available. Most people will not feel the need for one or even prefer no one else to be present. Offering a chaperone may be enough to reassure someone that one is not required. The response to this offer may also be of use in that it may prompt the discussion of how someone feels about being examined. If you find yourself avoiding or delaying a physical examination, this is a significant finding in its own right – what is it about a physical examination that is so difficult with *this* patient? Is it the patient's fear of what you might find – too terrible to be shown, so small or ugly that you might ridicule it (the vagina or penis), too young (emotionally) to be examined or a repeat of previous abuse?

Occasionally a physical examination can help the patient to talk about things that they would otherwise have concealed – as though taking off their clothes also helps to remove other barriers. Be an *active* observer during the physical examination and use the non-verbal clues just as much as in the history taking. Be purposeful and systematic in the examination. The patient should be quite clear about the normality or otherwise of the examination as you proceed and understand why you are doing each part. The examination may be routine for you but the patient can misunderstand unless you communicate the findings in the context of the problem.

You may find specific conditions like osteoarthritis of the hips causing difficulty with abduction of the legs, atrophic vulvovaginitis or reduction of peripheral pulses suggesting arteriosclerosis.

Some people will regard themselves as not being sexual because of illness or disability, or as being undesirable. There may be changes in relationships because of illness or disability. It is often difficult to switch from a caring role (especially if intimate personal needs are involved) to that of a lover. If you are not sure how to manage the sexual difficulties associated with these and other physical problems – you could look them up[10,11] or include this in your future learning.

Investigations for sexual problems

Be guided by the history. Investigations are occasionally prompted by the complaint of loss of desire but usually as a response to other indicators in the history.

Sometimes you need to do investigations so that the patient can consider causes other than physical ones. Be cautious in ascribing the cause of the sexual problem to any abnormality found. For example, a patient with pelvic inflammatory disease may have loss of desire because she believes her partner to have been unfaithful, not just because you have found chlamydia.

Female investigations might include the following tests:

- prolactin level – raised levels may be due to medical treatment or indicate a pituitary problem. A mildly raised level may not be significant. The test should be repeated if raised levels are recorded
- follicle stimulating hormone and luteinising hormone to establish whether a woman is menopausal (especially if the patient has had a hysterectomy or has amenorrhoea and is under 50 years of age) or has a pituitary problem
- thyroid hormone and thyroid stimulating hormone levels
- liver function tests (if drug or alcohol abuse is suspected)
- biochemical screen or full blood count (e.g. in complaints of fatigue to exclude physical illness such as diabetes, leukaemia or Addison's disease)
- ultrasound scan of the pelvic organs for elucidation or exclusion of abnormal findings
- laparoscopy if the history is suggestive of pelvic inflammatory disease or endometriosis.

You might do some of the blood tests listed above as part of the investigation of loss of desire or erectile dysfunction in men. Further discussion of men's sexual problems is in Chapter 8 on men's sexual health.

One of the difficulties in doing investigations is the interpretation of the results **3** of the tests. If there are minor abnormalities, the patient may become fixated on these as the 'cause' of the problem rather than looking at the whole picture. For example, although many men with diabetes suffer from erectile dysfunction, there may be contributory problems such as the devastation felt when a diag- nosis of a chronic disease is made, the bereavement feelings of loss of previous perceptions of good health, the impact on earning ability (e.g. in a heavy goods vehicle driver) and changes in the relationship.

If you are not the patient's GP and the results of tests are not normal, you need to consider how this information can be passed to the relevant personal medical attendant. Have you obtained informed consent from the patient to give this information to other health professionals?

Reasons for sexual problems

These include: **1**

- lack of knowledge
- lack or loss of desire
- dislike of sex

- poor performance or satisfaction
- medical conditions or medicines
- breakdown of relationship
- stress or tiredness.

Lack of knowledge

This is still surprisingly common. It may be due to being brought up in a family where sex was not mentioned. Sometimes a lack of knowledge can be due to abuse, or an unpleasant event, that makes the patient avoid sources of information.

Patients can borrow or buy factual books about sex, or watch factual films. Be cautious about recommending fiction or films showing sexual acts that may represent fantasies and not reality. Just as clothes are shown on tall, super-thin models, people paid to portray sexual acts tend not to be Mr or Mrs Average!

Lack or loss of desire

Many people complain about this when they have a lower level of sexual interest than their partner does. They often enjoy sex when they get going, but rarely think about it and do not approach their partner. It can be due to:

- myths about the roles of men and women
- fear of being found not to be good enough at sex – so it is avoided
- being too busy or preoccupied with other matters – common in couples who have children and jobs that keep them on the go all the time
- being ill, depressed or grieving – it is usual not to want sex if attention is focused on something else
- guilt about sexual activity – because of upbringing, religious beliefs or that they are letting someone else down
- fear – of pregnancy, or infection, or damage (common after a heart attack, operation or stroke)
- boredom – the same routine may be turning them off
- concentrating on the bad points of the partner instead of the reasons why they got together in the first place.

The first step towards sorting out the problem is to talk about when it started and to find out why the person might have a problem.

Loss of desire is the commonest sexual complaint in women, but is a spectrum of disorders. The complaint may have always been present. It may represent inhibition – a repression of sexual thoughts due to feelings of being too young (whatever the chronological age), too pure (sex is dirty or unsuitable in some way) or forbidden (by upbringing or religious taboo). It may represent a lack of compatibility between the expectations of the couple, either real or due to beliefs in myths.

Life events have a powerful effect on sexual functioning and sexual problems are more likely at critical times such as:

- beginning sexual life
- getting married
- having a baby
- having adolescents at home
- children leaving home
- losses – jobs, parents, health, youthfulness, opportunities, partners etc.
- chronic mental or physical illness
- moving into old age or what the person perceives as old age
- reminders of old psychological damage such as sexual or emotional abuse.

Some medical problems may cause loss of desire or make it more likely. Apart from the specific effects of the disease process itself, feeling unwell tends to focus attention on the illness rather than on pleasure and enjoyment of sexual activity.

Be cautious in laying the blame on medical problems – it may be a false clue.   **3**
Many people who are seriously or chronically ill will not be interested in sexual activity, but for others it is an important and essential reaffirmation of their love for each other even when terminally ill.

Looking at the circumstances of the difficulty for that couple or individual helps them to make sense of the situation and what they might do to modify or remedy the underlying causes. Sometimes the cause may be loss of attraction for, or even dislike of, the partner. If the health professional dislikes the partner from the description given, perhaps the patient does too! Relationship therapy may be an option for motivated couples, or sometimes the patient just needs to come to terms with the realisation that the partnership has to end. More often it is a combination of several small adjustments in attitudes, thought patterns, assumptions or behaviour that the individual or couple can make that helps the complainant towards a resolution or acceptance of the problem.

Lack of performance

Lack of orgasm is a more common complaint in women than in men. Orgasmic dysfunction in women is often linked to myths about the responsibility of the male partner to be able to produce the orgasm 'for the woman'. Fears or inhibitions about masturbation may have prevented a woman from discovering how to produce an orgasm herself, or she may have been unable to transfer this experience to heterosexual activity. Exploration of her own erotic areas, self-stimulation and better communication between partners during sexual arousal and intercourse can lead to a resolution unless psychological barriers protecting the patient from hidden fears are too great.

Vaginismus

Vaginismus is the *symptom* of a disorder in which spasm of the vaginal muscles prevents the penis entering the vagina or the penis can only be allowed in with pain or discomfort. Penetration may be impossible and the woman may be unable to:

- touch the vulva herself
- find any opening
- allow anyone else to touch
- allow anything inside.

She may sometimes be able to have a vaginal delivery after artificial insemination (i.e. something can come out even if not allowed in).

Secondary vaginismus has often been caused by the woman's experience of pain after infection, forced intercourse, a difficult delivery, imagined or real disfigurement after episiotomy, or any instrumentation in that area whether vaginal, urethral or rectal.

Primary vaginismus is usually due to fear and is similar to a panic disorder or phobia. This is rarely susceptible to an operation under anaesthetic to 'open it up', however tempting it may be to think in these mechanistic plumbing terms. Many women with minor problems can be helped with advice and learning how to explore their own vagina to remove the fear of the unknown. Others have a more complex phobia or fantasies that can take many months of therapy.[13] A physical barrier (e.g. an intact tough hymen or a vaginal septum) may also occasionally be present but may not necessarily be causative. You may wish to refer someone seeking more than simple help to a psychosexual therapist. A busy gynaecology outpatient clinic is not the best place for such help, unless the gynaecologist is known to have a special interest and expertise in such problems.

If a woman presents with vaginismus it is important to establish why she is asking for help.

If she only wants to have a baby, then she may only want to have sufficient help and advice to allow self-administered artificial insemination. She may not be able to permit vaginal examination by others and she will need sympathetic midwifery and obstetric assistance to proceed through pregnancy. Delivery may need to be by Caesarean section. Pressure from her religious or cultural circumstances may make her seek this path.

If, on the other hand, her desire is to have sexual intercourse with penile penetration, the outcome must be for her to be able to welcome her partner's penis inside her. A supportive therapist can facilitate gradual progression from self-exploration of the woman's own anatomy to insertion of small things like a fingertip or the smallest vaginal trainer. Vaginal trainers are sometimes called dilators. This unsuitable name often provokes a fearful response and is best avoided. They are available in graduated sizes and different colours such as pink or white. Some women will prefer to use the slightly more remote feeling of the trainer; others prefer the controllable feelings and feedback that they achieve with their own fingers. Offering a choice helps the woman to feel more in control of the penetration.

Sometimes progress is made rapidly and the woman will be able to go from feeling with one finger to two and then three, stretching the opening and discovering that it is not painful. Gaining the cooperation of the partner for the woman to follow on by controlling the insertion of the penis can lead rapidly to pleasurable penetrative intercourse.

Other women may have more problems. They may progress very slowly, avoiding using the trainer or finger for weeks until the fantasy or difficulty preventing them from trying is revealed and explored verbally. A woman may progress well with fingers or the trainers, but be unable to transfer her learning to penetration with the penis for other unspoken reasons, sometimes buried in her subconscious. Facing the fear may be just too great a challenge. Another source of disappointment is the partner who has previously enjoyed non-penetrative sexual activity, but has problems of his own about penetration. He may lose his erection faced with having to insert it inside the vagina, or avoid sexual activity altogether. Sometimes, the relationship founders once the woman becomes more assertive about her own sexual needs and desires. Perhaps the passive partner, that was so necessary when she could not have penetration, no longer suits her once she can.

Women who have progressed through all the stages of therapy to successful penile penetration may relapse after adverse circumstances. They are more likely to have vaginismus again if they have any painful condition of the vulva or vagina, such as after delivery or after an infection. They may need a 'top-up' of therapy but, provided their motivation for therapy was to achieve intercourse, they usually progress rapidly to a resolution of the difficulty. Those who do not, especially after delivery, may well have hidden the real reason for originally seeking therapy, or have developed other underlying relationship or psychological problems.

Vulval pain

Superficial vulval pain is common and has a multiplicity of possible underlying **2** factors:

- vulvitis or vulvovaginitis from infection or inflammation of the vulva and/or vagina
- vulval vestibulitis – with severe pain to the touch around the vulval vestibule at the entrance to the vagina
- vulvodynia – a condition of persisting pain of unknown aetiology, possibly related to post-viral infection sensitivity or psychological fears, that may overlap with vestibulitis
- urethritis from mechanical inflammation or infection
- atrophic vulvitis from lowered levels of oestrogen
- inadequate lubrication from low levels of oestrogen, anxiety or inadequate arousal
- irritants such as spermicides, detergents, scents, dyes or sweat.

Although the majority of women have short-lived symptoms, relieved by treatment of the underlying cause, a few continue to suffer considerable distress. Some resolve (after exclusion of infection) with graduated reducing doses of topical steroids, for others it may be part of a psychological defence, and a few remain 'medically unexplained' even after tertiary specialist referral and investigation.

Some women can be helped by the techniques described for vaginismus. Others **3** will need a combination of physical treatment and supportive therapy. For many women, just being believed that they have pain, in the absence of physical findings, is a relief in itself. Confirming to a partner that the health professional believes that the pain is real can improve the relationship if the partner has believed that the woman is avoiding sexual intercourse for other reasons. It is obviously important that the health professional does not collude with the woman in prolonging avoidance from intercourse and other causes for lack of penetration should always be explored.

The skin should be treated to make it less sensitive. This is usually done using a strong steroid combined with antibacterial and antifungal substances to reduce the inflammation, burning and swelling. Gradual reduction of the strength of the steroid cream prevents a rebound and thinning of the skin, and most people can reduce to occasional use of a mild steroid that is safe long term. Zinc oxide cream helps some women as zinc has been shown to reduce inflammation. A few women are helped by a combination of treatment to the skin and antifungal tablets. Xylocaine gel is a local anaesthetic gel that can be used short term if the pain is very great. However, it can cause allergic reactions if used long term.

The nerves can also be made less sensitive. Treatments, used in higher doses for depressive illness, can be used to slow down the rate at which the pain impulses pass along the nerve. Research has shown that chronic pain 'opens the pain gate', increasing the perception of pain. Treatments used successfully in many people are tricyclic antidepressants (e.g. amitryptiline) and specific serotonin re-uptake inhibitors (e.g. fluoxetine). Of course, having pain for a long time can be depressing and larger doses may be required for people with other symptoms of depression such as early morning waking or loss of pleasure in life.

Alternative sexual activity and plenty of comforting cuddles are very important. Most sufferers value support from a health professional or alternative practitioner. Many have found alternative therapies (acupuncture, herbal, homeopathy etc.) of value, although there is no good evidence for their effectiveness — so make sure they go to a reputable practitioner.

Sufferers have suggested other helpful treatments:

- Aveeno (oatmeal) baths — sit in the bath up to four times a day
- Indian teabags — warm and placed on the vulva or put in the bathwater
- aqueous cream as an emollient — if it is kept in the fridge it is more effective at cooling down the burning and can be used as often as needed
- a diet low in oxalates might help but the evidence for this is poor.

See the Appendix for a helpful website to recommend for patients, but warn them that people's experience of vulval pain can be very different.

Very occasionally the pain persists, and specialist referral may be arranged. A few people have surgery, but this is a last resort as it does leave a tender scar (although this may be preferable to what went before). It is important that both the psychological distress and the physical symptoms are treated together. The secondary vaginal spasm may still need to be treated even after the vulval pain has improved — and most people do improve with time.

Infertility

It is very stressful for a couple to be concentrating on having intercourse 'to order', whether they feel desire for intercourse or not. The investigations, the waiting and the disappointments all add to the lack of enjoyment in sexual activity. Some infertility may be secondary to lack of intercourse or non-consummation so that a good sexual history is essential right at the start. It is important that a couple undergoing investigations and treatment for infertility are encouraged to have sexual activity for enjoyment as well as procreation.

Hysterectomy and other operations

Hysterectomy for heavy bleeding usually improves sexual functioning,[14] but patients often complain that they are given insufficient information about sexual activity afterwards. Patients who had a bulky uterus may find they have altered sensation and need to change positions afterwards to achieve the same stimulation. Quite a few women (and their partners) are fearful of doing some damage to the scar afterwards, or that the vagina will not be long enough to contain the penis. Factual information hand-outs promote good sexual functioning after the operation.

These basic principles apply to other operations in that area, but there may be complications from tender scar tissue after a repair for vaginal prolapse or vulval surgery, cancer fears or lack of oestrogen after removal of the ovaries.

Pregnancy and childbirth

There is a reduction in the frequency of intercourse, and interest and satisfaction with sexual activity, over the course of a pregnancy. There is a wide variation between couples in sexual responsiveness, enjoyment and level of activity. Sexual problems after delivery are common, but a survey showed that only about 15% reported discussing them with a health professional.[15] At three months 58% had experienced painful intercourse, 39% vaginal dryness (this is especially likely if breast-feeding) and 44% loss of sexual desire. By eight to nine months after delivery about a quarter to a third of the women were still experiencing some problems.

Myths about sexual activity

Some of the myths about sex that people believe in (even when they deny it) are listed below:

- men are always ready for sex
- men do not show or talk about emotions

- a lover always knows how their partner feels without having to ask or be told
- men should always take the lead, initiate and orchestrate sexual activity
- it is a man's job to satisfy the woman and bring her to orgasm
- all physical contact between a couple leads to sexual activity
- sexual activity is always penile penetration of the vagina leading to ejaculation
- sexual activity should be natural and spontaneous, never planned or set up
- failure to achieve erection or orgasm is a disaster and means that the person does not love/desire the partner
- everyone should be able to have successful sexual intercourse without practising or learning how to do it better
- both members of a couple will always feel ready to have sex at the same time.

Referral

Ideally, referral onwards occurs when the patient and the health professional agree to seek a specialist opinion, or for more specialist investigations or treatment.

Sometimes, patients will just ask for a referral because they do not want to discuss their sexual dysfunction with you. This can be because of embarrassment, fear of judgemental attitudes (their own as well as yours), fears about confidentiality or because they feel you are not the right person to help them. Make sure you explore what they are expecting from specialist referral — a magic wand is not available!

However, it is still important to establish what the problem is and who is the most relevant professional to help them. You can only refer for expert help if you know who the experts are. Meeting and talking with the staff from the range of facilities in your area is the best way of being able to discuss with patients who would be the best choice for their particular difficulty.

References

1 Sickle MA and Rosenstock H (1999) Taking a sexual history: which questions to ask. *The Female Patient* **24**: 33.
2 Merrill JM, Laux LF and Thonby JI (1990) Why doctors have difficulty with sex histories. *Southern Medical Journal* **83**: 616.
3 Dunn KM, Croft PR and Hackett G (1998) Sexual problems: a study of the prevalence and need for healthcare in the general population. *Family Practice* **15**: 519–24.

4 Wellings K, Field J, Johnson AM and Wadsworth J (1994) *Sexual Behaviour in Britain*. Penguin Books, London.

5 National Survey of Sexual Attitudes and Lifestyles (NATSAL 2000), www.qb.soc. surrey.ac.uk/surveys/natsal/nssalintro.htm.

6 Johnson AM, Mercer C, Evans B *et al.* (2001) Sexual behaviour in Britain: partnerships, practice and HIV risk behaviours. *Lancet* **358**: 1835–42.

7 Wellings K, Nanchatal K, MacDowell W *et al.* (2001) Sexual behaviour in Britain: early sexual behaviour. *Lancet* **358**: 1843–50.

8 Fenton KA, Korovessis C, Johnson AM *et al.* (2001) Sexual behaviour in Britain: reported sexually transmitted infections and prevalent genital Chlamydia trachomatis infection. *Lancet* **358**: 1851–54.

9 Chambers R, Wakley G, Field S and Ellis S (2002) *Appraisal for the Apprehensive*. Radcliffe Medical Press, Oxford.

10 Skrine R and Montford H (eds) (2001) *Psychosexual Medicine: an introduction*. Arnold Publishing, London.

11 Cooper E and Guillebaud J (1999) *Sexuality and Disability: a guide for everyday practice*. Radcliffe Medical Press, Oxford.

12 Dunn KM, Croft PR and Hackett G (1999) Association of sexual problems with social, psychological and physical problems in men and women: a cross-sectional population study. *Journal of Epidemiology and Community Health* **53**: 144–8.

13 Valins L (1988) *Vaginismus: understanding and overcoming the blocks to intercourse*. Ashgrove Press, Bath.

14 Ferroni P and Deeble J (1996) Women's subjective experience of hysterectomy. *Australian Health Review* **19**: 40–55.

15 Barrett G, Pendry E, Peacock J *et al.* (2000) Women's sexual health after childbirth. *British Journal of Obstetrics and Gynaecology* **107**: 186–95.

5

Sexual health screening and investigation

What is screening?

Screening is a programme directed towards the detection of a specific disease **1** or condition in a target group: for example, cervical cancer in women of a particular age group, raised blood pressure in adults of a particular age group, or infections in people without symptoms. Screening makes use of tests that can be applied rapidly to apparently well persons. The tests are used to distinguish between those who probably have the condition and those who probably do not.

What is the difference between screening and investigation?

Both use tests, often the same tests, to determine whether an individual has a **1** certain condition or disease. The difference is in the populations to which those individuals belong. Testing individuals who have no symptoms, or who have a low risk of the condition or disease, is screening. Investigation is the testing of those who have symptoms or a high risk of the disease.

The predictive value of tests

Investigation and screening may overlap. For example, if a woman aged 23 years **2** presents to you with bleeding after intercourse between her periods, you might want to take a cervical swab for chlamydia testing and a cervical smear for cervical cytology. The prevalence of chlamydia in the population to which she belongs is high, perhaps 10–12% in her age group. If she has additional risk factors, such as several changes of partner in the last 12 months, she is at quite high risk of having a chlamydial infection. You might regard taking a swab for chlamydia as an *investigation*.

She is much less likely to have an abnormal cervical smear. If she has had a recent screening test, it might be reasonable not to include this. If she has not had a recent satisfactory test, offer to do a cervical smear as a screening test.

A *positive chlamydial test* would confirm your suspicions, i.e. the positive predictive value (PPV) of the test is high, but a negative test would not entirely allay them. A *negative cervical smear* would confirm your supposition that the cause is not cervical cancer, i.e. the negative predictive value (NPV) is high.

If this woman is aged 53 years and presents with vaginal bleeding after intercourse, your priorities will be different. She is much less likely to have chlamydia, as she is much less likely to have had more than one recent sexual partner or to have had sexual intercourse with men who have had several partners. Cervical cancer becomes more common as women become older, so she is more likely to have this. You might think about *screening* for chlamydia if she has had a recent change of partner and taking a cervical smear as an *investigation* indicated by the clinical history. (She might have other causes such as post-menopausal vulval or vaginal atrophy, or abnormalities of the endometrium.)

A *positive chlamydial test* would surprise you and you might decide to repeat the test to confirm it, i.e. the NPV is higher. A *negative cervical smear test* would not entirely reassure you, especially if she has not had a previous test. That is, the PPV is higher. You might repeat the test to increase the accuracy of the result or arrange a different examination like a culposcopic examination of the cervix.

So:

- if the disease is common, the PPV of the test is higher
- if the disease is rare, the NPV is higher
- PPV is the proportion of those with a positive test who have the disease
- NPV is the proportion of those with a negative test who do not have the disease.

Sensitivity and specificity of tests

The sensitivity of a test is the proportion of those in that population who have the disease who test positive. For example, If 100 people have the disease, and only 85 test positive, the sensitivity is 85%.

The specificity of a test is the proportion of the population without the disease who test negative. The specificity of a new test has to be determined by comparison with another test (or tests) that correctly determines that the disease is absent.

These characteristics do not depend on the frequency of the disease.

Characteristics of a screening test

Screening test characteristics can be illustrated using a two by two chart.

2

		Screen result	
		Negative	Positive
Disease present	No	A	B
	Yes	C	D

A = the number of people who do not have the disease and test negative. If the disease is relatively uncommon, the majority of people will be in this group and will be minimally affected by having a screening test by, for example, the inconvenience or personal costs.

B = the number of people who do not have the disease but have a positive screening test. This is a false positive test. They will be adversely affected by having the screening, largely because of anxiety and follow-up diagnostic tests that may have further adverse effects. If the disease is uncommon, this will be the second largest group.

C = the number of people who do have the disease but have a negative test result. This is a false negative test. If the disease is uncommon this will be the smallest group, but they are potentially adversely affected by, for example, not being treated early, or by being falsely reassured so that they or their medical attendants ignore subsequent symptoms or signs of illness.

D = the number of people who have the disease and have a positive result. These are the main beneficiaries of the screening, provided the treatment available is effective.

False results

The false positive rate = 1 minus the specificity = the proportion of disease-free subjects testing positive by the screening test. This is usually easy to calculate as subjects with a positive result are usually thoroughly investigated.

3

The false negative rate = 1 minus the sensitivity = the proportion of subjects with the disease missed by the screening test. This may be impossible to determine in practice. People who test negative are not usually investigated any further. Estimates are often made by assuming that the persons who develop the disease within a set time after screening were falsely negative − but they may have developed the disease anew during that time.

If the limitations of the screening procedure have not been made clear or there are perceived high false positive rates, this will affect the acceptability of the screening – as it has done in cervical cytology screening. Public perception has often been to conclude that it is not worth having a test when they think that the results are unreliable.[1,2]

Prevention by screening

The population in which the screening is carried out should be one in which **1** the condition is relatively frequent, significant and can be identified before it causes adverse effects. It should be susceptible to treatment, and the treatment should be available in the region in which the population is situated.

It is harmful to introduce screening if there is no prospect of adequate treatment.

Primary and secondary prevention

In clinical situations such as primary care, the terms primary and secondary **2** prevention are used in specific ways (which differ from those used in public health):

- primary prevention is targeting individuals who are at risk of developing a condition and screening them before they develop disease or adverse effects from that condition
- secondary prevention is aimed at people who already have a condition and preventing further adverse effects.

For example, pregnant women are tested to see if they have antibodies to syphilis. If they have, they may have been infected previously (although a few other conditions produce false positive results). The aim is to prevent further complications in the mother (secondary prevention) and to prevent transmission to the infant (primary prevention).

In investigating suspected conditions, health professionals often choose tests for their sensitivity and specificity. They often underestimate the importance of the predictive value when transferring the test from investigation to screening. When it is very important not to miss a diagnosis, we choose a test with high sensitivity for our investigation.

In screening it is often important not to create false positives because of the serious consequences of a positive diagnosis, so we may want a test with a higher specificity. To achieve this aim we may have to accept a test that has a lower sensitivity than the alternative test that may worry people unnecessarily about a false positive result.[3]

Public health definitions of prevention

Primary prevention targets society as a whole, no matter what the risk is to the   **3**
individual. Wearing a condom when first starting intercourse is always recommended. It does not take into account whether you are at high risk (starting a sexual relationship with someone who has had multiple sexual partners) or low risk (a couple starting a sexual relationship who have never had sexual intercourse).

Primary care is not usually involved in the decisions about instituting primary prevention programmes that are taken centrally by governments, but may be active in promoting the principles or carrying out the process of primary prevention, such as immunisation programmes.

Secondary prevention identifies individuals who either have an increased risk, or are in the early stages, of a disease that can be treated effectively. It may target large groups of the population as in cervical screening or blood pressure screening.

Tertiary prevention is concerned with reducing the occurrence, the recurrence or the effects of a previously diagnosed disease or condition. An example would be avoiding oestrogen-containing contraceptives in someone who previously had hypertension while taking this type of pill, and monitoring the blood pressure at intervals to determine if it reached levels requiring treatment.

What harm can screening do?

Screening without proof of benefit is really experimentation and not screening.   **1**
Before using a screening test ask:

- Is there evidence from randomised research trials that supports the use of this test for screening?
- Is the potential person suitable for screening (e.g. without symptoms)?
- Is this the right time to screen this person (e.g. at a stage when a test will identify the condition)?
- Are you sure that there are adequate procedures in place to follow up the person if the test is positive?

Whilst screening has the potential to save lives or improve quality of life through early diagnosis of serious conditions, it is not a foolproof process. Screening can reduce the risk of developing a condition or its complications but it cannot offer a guarantee of protection. This is often not understood by, or explained adequately to, the population being offered screening. In any screening programme there are false positive results (wrongly reported as having the condition) and false negative results (wrongly reported as *not* having the condition). If there were likely to be too many false positives, it would be irresponsible to introduce a screening programme as too many people would be subjected to medical procedures they did not need. They would not only have the screening test but also further diagnostic tests and possibly unnecessary treatment.

2

Considering the harm that breast screening can do

The risk of a woman aged 50–60 years developing breast cancer is two per 1000 a year or 2% over a decade (20 out of 1000 women). Currently the anticipated 10-year survival rate for clinically detected breast cancer in the absence of screening is about 75%. Therefore, we can expect five deaths per 1000 women from breast cancer over this period (75% of 20).[4] The relative risk reduction for screening applies to these five women. A realistic estimate of the current effects of treatment might be the saving of one life. Therefore, one in 1000 women stand to benefit from a decade of screening whilst 999 women bear the cost both in monetary and personal terms.

3

Many women with non-cancerous changes on mammography will be recalled for biopsy. There always has to be a fine balance between these opposing needs, to identify all the cancers whilst protecting women without cancer from false alarms and unnecessary invasive procedures. Even when the screening programme is working at its best, many women will have false positive results for every one cancer truly detected.

Surgery itself has its risks and harms but there is also the difficulty of deciding what is abnormal from the biopsy samples taken. The public and many health professionals tend to assume that a pathologist can make a clear distinction between cancer and non-cancer, but it is not that clear-cut. There is a whole range of abnormalities of uncertain significance and unknown natural history. If screening picks up a cancer, the woman may live with the diagnosis of cancer for longer than if she had not been screened and the cancer was picked up only when it became obvious. In other words, even when this screening does pick up a cancer the woman's life may not be extended. Worse still, she may be subjected to an operation, perhaps a mastectomy, and a label of 'breast cancer' for a condition that would never have affected her health or life expectancy. This type of 'breast cancer' (such as low-grade ductal carcinoma *in situ*) is of unknown significance and may well not progress to clinical significance.

The radiation to which the breast tissue is exposed may also be harmful in its own right. We know that X-ray exposure increases the risk of cancer. So a balance between the risks of this method of screening and the results obtained must be made. In some affluent societies women are encouraged to purchase frequent screening in the misplaced belief that this will increase their chances of 'preventing cancer'. Screening does not 'prevent cancer', it will only pick up what is already there and there is only benefit if the test is accurate and the treatment successful in removing the cancer. They might be increasing their risks of developing cancer by more frequent mammography.

Similarly, there have been calls for mammography for younger age groups. Not only is breast cancer much less common in the under 50 year olds, the natural history and types of cancer are different and the more dense breast tissue less suitable for accurate identification of small cancers. Two summary overviews of breast screening[5,6] were unable to show any benefit for screening women under 50 years of age.

It is a difficult balance to make and arguments will continue unless screening is only introduced with clear evidence of benefits exceeding the harms.

Screening for chlamydia

Pilot studies are currently investigating this for effectiveness. The principles for utilising screening in this scenario provide a useful example (see Box 5.1).

2

Box 5.1 General principles to consider when introducing screening of well people for illnesses or infections with special regard to chlamydia

- *Is the condition important?* Chlamydia is an important cause of infertility, ectopic pregnancy, salpingitis, chronic pelvic pain and morbidity.
- *Is the natural history well understood?* Seventy to eighty per cent of women have cervical infections with no symptoms, but it is not clear how many have a risk of ascending infections in the absence of precipitating factors such as instrumentation of the uterus.
- *Is there a recognisable early stage?* Screening tests can identify infection when no symptoms are present.
- *Is there a suitable test?* The nucleic acid amplification tests are more sensitive and specific than the previous enzyme immunoassay tests and

can be done on urine as well as swabs. Blood tests are not useful as they tell you only if someone has ever had the infection (and possibly got rid of it), not whether they have it currently.

- *Is the test acceptable?* Urine tests are more acceptable than cervical or urethral swabs. Self-taken swabs have also been shown to be useful and acceptable in some groups.
- *At what intervals should the test be repeated?* Unknown – and may depend on the accuracy and completeness of contact tracing and treatment, and on social factors like change of sexual partner or monogamy.
- *Are there adequate facilities for the diagnosis and treatment?* No – primary care health professionals do not generally have sufficient time or skills, GUM clinics could not cope with the number of referrals of people with positive tests and the laboratories have insufficient capacity and resources to carry out the tests. Instigating a publicity campaign about chlamydia (so that greater numbers of people self-refer themselves for screening) without increasing the facilities for screening, further testing for confirmation and for treatment would cause collapse of the present, already overstretched arrangements.
- *Is treatment at an early stage of more benefit than treatment at a later stage?* Definitely – infection can easily be eradicated in the early stages before structural damage occurs.
- *Are the chances of physical and psychological harm less than the chances of benefit?* This depends on how the test is presented, people's feelings about stigmatisation (having a 'sexually transmitted infection') and public knowledge about the condition.

- *Can the cost be balanced against the benefits the service provides, versus other opportunity costs and benefits?* Unknown as yet – early pilot studies from Merseyside[7] and Southampton[8] showed much higher prevalence of infection and higher costs for the counselling time and number of tests performed than expected. Further pilots at 10 sites are ongoing.

Guidelines for screening for chlamydia

You may already have local guidelines for screening for chlamydia. Compare these with some other guidelines available from the Royal College of Physicians[9] or the Scottish Intercollegiate Guideline Network (SIGN) guidelines.[10] You can read about setting up your own guidelines that might be part of a development plan in your workplace in the book *Sexual Health Matters in Primary Care.*[11]

3

Ethical considerations of chlamydia screening

Young women are being targeted for screening. This may stigmatise the women as being 'the cause' of a STI. The current screening proposals pay scant regard to the role of young men in the spread of this STI. There are difficulties in tracing and treating the partners of the women identified as positive and the health service needs to set up new procedures.[12] For example, women presenting for termination of pregnancy are 'screened' for chlamydia (or should be). They often leave hospital before the results of the tests are known, having been treated empirically as though they have the infection. Women with positive results are difficult to contact later (they usually want to forget about what has happened and have no contact with the hospital). Their partners are not treated and some studies have shown that those given antibiotic treatment in hospital and then followed up often become rapidly reinfected.[13] Communication of results between the providers of health services can be poor. Those performing the tests may have not thought through how to ensure that the results can be passed to the patient and the patient's usual healthcare provider in a secure manner to ensure confidentiality, and in a reliable way to ensure the treatment of the woman and her partner.

Screening for STIs

If a person has been exposed to one STI, they may have acquired others. It is usual to screen, or investigate, for all the common STIs when a person is attending a GUM clinic. The degree to which each test can be said to be screening or investigation depends on the sexual history and the symptoms and signs. Many people attend for screening with no symptoms, but with a fear that they may have contracted a STI because of their sexual behaviour. The confidentiality of testing at a GUM clinic helps to encourage people to come forward for testing, but the stigma of attending, together with the inconvenience and perceived discomfort of the tests, are disincentives.

In general practice, it is usual to be more selective. Tests for STIs are usually only done as investigations when the degree of probability of infection is raised from the history or clinical picture.

Informed consent

Any test that is done must be carried out with informed consent. It is unethical to do a test if the person involved does not understand the implications of a test that may result in a positive result. After the publicity about HIV infection, many people attended asking for tests, but without having thought through what they would do given the result. Those requesting a test did not usually understand that there was a period between infection and seroconversion (appearance of antibodies in the blood) when the test would be negative. If their sexual behaviour was such to put them at risk, then the primary consideration was an alteration in attitude to that risk and perhaps more general screening for other STIs as well. If the test results were negative, would this mean those individuals continuing to put themselves (and others) at risk of STIs? How often would they want to repeat the test?

A large number of people do not want their GP to have the information about their HIV status (or other results of STI testing). Confidentiality and stigma are still problems for people with HIV, which will increase if the counselling and testing for HIV is moved into general practice as envisaged by the *National Strategy for Sexual Health and HIV*.[14]

Which STIs do you screen for?

GUM clinics usually have a set protocol for screening and dealing with the results. Some general practices will have looked at this and provided guidelines, for example for the investigation and management of complaints of vaginal discharge, but it would be more appropriate for a request for *screening* to be referred to a GUM clinic. If you cannot do it well, it is better not to offer it as incomplete screening will mislead people and lull them into a false sense of security.

An example of the tests that would be offered to someone seeking screening is given below and is taken from the website for genitourinary medicine (see website list in the Appendix). These tests would be offered to someone who has been subjected to a sexual assault or rape (under the strict rules of keeping the evidence chain documented and clear). The guidelines suggest:

- swabs for testing for gonorrhoea and chlamydia
- slides for microscopy for yeasts, bacterial vaginosis (BV) and *Trichomonas vaginalis* (TV)
- blood for syphilis serology and a serum sample to save. Hepatitis B, HIV and, if indicated, hepatitis C testing should be offered as the patient may have a pre-existing risk of infection. If testing is not indicated, the sample should be saved to clarify the timing of any subsequent seroconversion (i.e. the appearance of antibody markers for these infections).

Screening of pregnant women

The policy for screening pregnant women for infection is a subject for hot debate in the UK.

A report in 1999 gave information about testing from information responses from 140 of the 192 UK obstetric units.[15] Universal screening for syphilis was being carried out, but a few units were considering stopping this. Testing for hepatitis B was offered to all women in just under half the units, with selective screening being offered in most of the others. There was a lack of consistency between policy (to screen) and practice (actually screening). The selection of women regarded as at risk was not consistent in units where selective screening was offered. The responsibility for following up test results was often unclear and infants were not always fully immunised even when their risk had been established. It was clear from this report that clear policies and systems for following up results were needed to ensure that screening was worthwhile.

Current research suggests that the strongest predictor of uptake rates for antenatal HIV testing appears to be the attitude of the midwife offering the test. Some midwives feel that the time available for the explanation of the test implications is insufficient to be able to obtain informed consent. Others hold a nihilistic view of HIV testing and treatment options – feeling that if a woman learns about her HIV status, that she will be receiving a death sentence for her and her child. Others are enthusiastic promoters of the test and encourage women to have it to try to reduce the transmission of infection to the infants.

Anonymous testing for HIV is not screening. It is monitoring the prevalence of HIV in that community. Testing without follow-up of positive results and arrangements for treatment is not screening. You might discuss with others the ethics of anonymous testing.

It has also been suggested that pregnant women should be screened for bacterial vaginosis. However, the natural history of BV infection is poorly understood, and further research is required to establish whether this is indeed a significant infection in pregnancy. It is possible that treatment of BV early in pregnancy could prevent early labour or reduce the number of stillbirths; however there are still unknown factors to establish, such as the rates of reinfection after treatment.

Hepatitis C screening

France introduced screening for hepatitis C in 1999–2000. This national campaign was launched with media campaigns and targeted information for health professionals. A free-phone information and advice number was provided. The prevalence of hepatitis C antibodies (HCV Ab) was around 1.1% in the population in France.

Some have advocated introducing this in the UK with others suggesting that it should be a more targeted investigation. One study in the UK found that the prevalence of HCV Ab was around 5% in those who had been found to have persistently raised liver enzymes, compared to 0.44% in blood donors. Another study of pregnant women offered testing at an inner-city London hospital found a hepatitis C prevalence of 0.8%, that is eight out of every 1000 women. This study found that offering testing was acceptable to the women, and most (73%) of the women with positive results did not have obvious risk factors such as drug abuse.

You might look for these articles and others on this controversy by doing a search on the National electronic Library of Medicine (see the website list in the Appendix). You can enter the terms 'screening and hepatitis' to find these articles and at least 17 others!

Cervical cytology screening

General principles to consider in cervical cytology screening are listed in Box 5.2.   **2**

Box 5.2   General principles to consider in cervical cytology screening

- *Is the condition important?* Approximately 3000 new cases of cervical cancer are diagnosed each year in England and Wales, leading to about 1200 deaths.
- *Is the natural history well understood?* No. Although mortality has been declining over the last 20 years, and the decline has accelerated since the introduction of screening in 1987, it would not now be ethical to randomise some women to a 'no-treatment' arm to see what happens to early abnormalities. We do not know how many of these early abnormalities might disappear without treatment.
- *Is there a recognisable early stage?* Screening tests can identify abnormal cells, but it is not known how often they may become cancerous. The progression of some abnormal cells into a pre-cancerous condition is thought to take between 10 and 15 years.
- *Is there a suitable test?* The current screening test is based on taking a sample of cells from the cervix with a wooden or plastic shaped spatula. The material collected is spread on a glass slide and sprayed with fixative. Specially trained cytologists examine the slide for abnormal cells. There are relatively high numbers of slides that are inadequate for examination because the cells are obscured by debris or blood, or are too thick or thin. Fatigue by cytologists is a significant cause of failure to avoid false negative or false positive results. The newer liquid-based cytology (see below) has a much lower rate of inadequate slides and clearer, more easily read slides with the potential for automated slide examination.

- *Is the test acceptable?* Most women endure the procedure for the perceived gain. Others will refuse, especially if they have lost faith in the procedure to protect them from false results. Coverage of the population is low in some socio-economic groups (often those at higher risk) and in some ethnic minority groups. See below for suggestions on how to increase uptake.
- *At what intervals should the test be repeated?* Screening at between three and five-year intervals provides the best chance of picking up abnormal cells. Decreasing the interval to less than three years increases the pick-up rate only slightly in those with a previous negative test. Some authorities suggest that screening should be every three years initially until two or three negative results have been obtained, then five-yearly.
- *Are there adequate facilities for the diagnosis and treatment?* No – there are often long waits for further investigation by colposcopy* and/or treatment. This increases anxiety and fear, especially as many women think that they have cancer rather than 'early warning cells'.
- *Is treatment at an early stage of more benefit than treatment at a later stage?* About half of the women who present with late-stage cervical cancer have never had a cervical smear. It does appear that early treatment of abnormal cells reduces the risk of later cervical cancer, but this may be at the cost of overtreatment of many who might not require any treatment if left alone.
- *Are the chances of physical and psychological harm less than the chances of benefit?* This depends on how the test is presented, public knowledge about the condition and procedures and how results are communicated. A study showed that use of the words 'early warning cells' reduced women's fear of having cancer when told they had a positive cervical smear result.[16]
- *Can the cost be balanced against the benefits the service provides, versus other opportunity costs and benefits?* There are no direct studies that give clear results about the cost-effectiveness of cervical screening. The introduction of screening was a triumph of hope (that cervical cancer could be prevented) over the evidence at the time. New efforts to determine the cost-effectiveness of introducing liquid-based cytology, or to target specific higher-risk groups (such as those with human papilloma virus [HPV] types 16 and 18) are under way.

---

* Colposcopy is the examination of the cervix with a high-powered lens. The picture is often projected onto a television screen so that the patient can see the area herself, and for training purposes. The cervix is painted with dilute acetic acid. This shows up inflammatory areas as white (aceto-white), so that biopsies or treatment can be targeted to those areas.

Further information on cervical screening

You could look at the NICE recommendations which contrast the present **3** arrangements for screening with the proposals for liquid-based cytology – see the NICE website or the links from the National electronic Library of Medicine website.

Liquid-based cytology

This method of screening for cervical cancer is being looked at in current pilot **3** studies. The sample is collected from the cervix in the same way, but using a special plastic broom-like device which is swept over the transitional zone five times to collect cellular material. The broom is rinsed in a vial of preservative. The vial is mixed in the laboratory and treated to remove unwanted material by an automated process. The remaining suspension of cells can be stained and the prepared slide looks much clearer for examination. The automation of the slide examination is also under trial. The proportion of inadequate smears (and subsequent repeat tests required) is greatly reduced.

The liquid suspension of cells can also be examined for the presence of HPV types 16 and 18 that have been shown to be associated with the development of cervical cancer. If this technique proves more accurate than the previous method, and can be combined with typing of HPV infections, it may permit the development of more selective follow-up and treatment.

There are even suggestions that the immunisation of populations with vaccines against HPV 16 and 18 will eliminate the need for screening (pilot studies are underway at present) – but that looks rather optimistic in the short term!

How to increase uptake of screening

Motivation

You might divide people into two main groups: **2**

- those who are motivated to find out how to prevent themselves becoming ill
- others who believe that what happens to them is 'fate'.

In practice most people fall between the two groups. People add in to their belief system information about the relative risks and benefits of having tests and early treatment. For cervical cytology, people are generally poorly informed and often agree to the test to please the nurse or doctor. Generally, the more control people believe they have over life events (even when unrealistic), the more likely they are to participate in screening. Being more open about the advantages and disadvantages of cervical screening enables people to take their own decisions.

Vulnerability

Many women do not believe that they are personally at risk and require more factual information about what is known about the natural history of the cancer. They think that their sexual lifestyle has protected them against developing cervical cancer. For example, they may think that the test is only for those who have had multiple partners, or that they do not need a test if they cease sexual activity.

Seriousness

Cancer is greatly feared and generally regarded as a death sentence. The fear (of what might be there) has to be balanced against the hope that treatment will prevent the development of cancer. Giving results in an insensitive way, delays for investigation and treatment, and lack of knowledge that 'early warning cells' are not cancer cells, increase the level of anxiety.

Costs

Costs include difficulties finding the time and the costs of travel and loss of earnings in attending for an internal examination, anxiety about being examined, especially by a doctor and even more by a male doctor (female nurses are preferred by many), and the embarrassment of that private part of the body being exposed to view.

Fear of the unknown

Many women attend without invitation, often after discussing the test with others such as a granddaughter or friend. More use of peer advisors and 'expert

patients' might improve uptake, but confidentiality problems may limit their
usefulness. The quality of their advice and their expertise as communicators
might also cause difficulties.

Present state of cervical screening in England[17]

A bulletin from the Department of Health describes the findings from the   **2**
computerised call and recall programme for cervical screening in England.[17]
Eighty-four per cent of women between 20 and 64 years had a result within the
last five years, similar results to each year since 1995. (In 1984 only just over
40% of women were being screened.) A total of 3.8 million women were
screened, most after a computerised call, and laboratories examined approximately 4.4 million smears. At laboratory level there was wide variation in the
percentage distribution of results, in particular in the proportion reported as
'borderline'. Separate reports are issued for Scotland, Wales and Northern
Ireland with similar results.

What do the laboratory reports mean for the health professional and the patient?

- *Severe dyskaryosis*: women are referred immediately for further investigation   **2**
  by colposcopy usually involving biopsies and perhaps removal of that area.
- *Moderate dyskaryosis*: women are referred immediately for colposcopy.
- *Mild dyskaryosis or borderline changes*: women are usually recalled for an early
  repeat of the test.

The correlation is poor between the smear appearance and the results from
colposcopy, or from biopsies. Warn women that the results from colposcopy
give a much better idea of what degree of abnormality is present. The abnormality may be much less or even absent, or occasionally worse.

Blood pressure screening

Most people do not think of measuring blood pressure as screening. It is a   **1**
good screening test − quick and easy to apply to large numbers of people with
no symptoms. A consistently raised level is a good marker for later disease and
will identify those with higher risk factors for conditions such as myocardial

infarction and stroke. The problems arise once a raised level has been established. It is difficult to persuade people to take medication when they do not feel ill, and who often feel less well on the medication than they did before!

Screening for hypertension

It is important that this simple test is carried out carefully. Labelling someone as hypertensive using inaccurate, unserviced or uncalibrated equipment, or using poor techniques, is bad screening with long-term adverse effects. Many audits of blood pressure recording have highlighted errors of technique or faulty equipment. You might look at the section on potential errors in measuring blood pressure in *Cardiovascular Disease Matters in Primary Care*.[17]

2

Screening for an increased risk of thrombosis (thrombophilia)

In our present state of knowledge about the factors leading to an increased risk of thrombosis, this cannot be justified. Although factor V Leiden is the most commonly identified hereditary disorder associated with venous thrombophilia, previously unknown thrombophilic genes are gradually being identified and a negative test does not rule out a hereditable condition. That is, the tests only give a positive predictive value, not a negative predictive value (which would be more useful for screening).

2

The National Screening Committee reported in June 2001 after organising a workshop on the use of family history or genetic markers to identify a high-risk group. They agreed a policy on genetic screening for inherited thrombophilia:

1 *Women considering oral contraception.* Advise women with a history of venous thrombosis to seek alternative methods of contraception if possible and counsel them about the level of risk. There is no evidence to support screening of such women for genetic mutations.
2 *Women of child-bearing age.* There is no evidence to support screening of women before conception for genetic predisposition to thrombophilia with the objective of reducing the risk of venous thrombosis in pregnancy.
3 *Women considering hormone replacement therapy.* Advise women with a history of venous thrombosis about the risk of hormone replacement therapy and about alternative interventions. There is no evidence to support screening of such women for genetic mutations.

4 *Familial cascade screening.* There is some evidence to support the systematic identification of the relatives of individuals with some forms of inherited thrombophilia and this should be managed through appropriate specialist clinics. This has obvious implications for confidentiality within family groups.

The National Screening Committee agreed to review the evidence by 2004 at the latest. You can look at the report of the workshop from the National electronic Library of Medicine website (see website list in the Appendix). Other reports about screening for common and less common disorders are also available on this site.

Screening for prostate cancer

Prostate cancer differs from many other cancers in the body in that small deposits of cancer within the prostate are very common. About one-third of men over the age of 50 years have a small focus of cancer within their prostate and nearly all men over the age of 80 years will have a small focus of prostate cancer. In the elderly particularly, these cancers grow very slowly and may never cause any problems. In other cases the cancer can grow rapidly and spread to other parts of the body, particularly the bones.

At present in the UK the decision not to introduce a population screening programme for prostate cancer has been made. The main reason for this was that the prostate-specific antigen (PSA) test has limited accuracy and could lead to a positive result for those without the disease. Follow-up procedures with side-effects of impotency and incontinence could cause unnecessary harm to healthy individuals. Medical opinion is divided about how to treat the disease and varies from 'watchful waiting' to radical surgery.

PSA levels increase with age and with other conditions of the prostate such as infection or the non-cancerous condition, benign prostatic hypertrophy (BPH). If there are symptoms a PSA test (i.e. used as an investigation) may be useful as part of the assessment to determine whether someone should be referred for a specialist opinion.

Men with early prostate cancer are unlikely to have any symptoms as these only occur when the cancer is large enough to put pressure on the urethra or disturb bladder function. Many older men have enlargement of the prostate due to non-cancerous BPH.

The symptoms of BPH and prostate cancer are similar and may include difficulty in passing urine, passing urine more frequently than usual (especially at night) and blood in the urine. The majority of men with these symptoms do not have prostate cancer. As prostate cancer is often a slow-growing cancer and symptoms may not occur for many years, even significant cancers may cause no urinary symptoms and the first symptoms may be pain in the back, hips or pelvis caused by the cancer spreading to the bones.

The main blood test for prostate cancer is the PSA test. This measures the level of PSA in a man's blood but is not a perfect guide. About 10 in 100 men who have prostate cancer do not have raised levels of PSA. Two-thirds of men who have raised levels of PSA, at the usual cut-off level, do not have prostate cancer. The PSA test cannot distinguish between men who have slow-growing prostate cancer and those who have a more aggressive disease. There are different PSA tests in use, and there can be up to 30% difference between the various types of tests and between the different laboratories that process them. This confuses health professionals and patients who find these variations complicate the assessment and decision-making process.

Research and pilot studies are underway to try to establish what cut-off point for a raised PSA level would be useful for screening. The test is really not a good enough one to lend itself to screening in people with no symptoms. It is only helpful if considerably raised in someone with symptoms of prostatic enlargement.

Screening for prostate cancer has aroused fierce emotions. Much in demand by **3** consumer groups, the PSA test is not, however, a reliable indicator of the presence of cancer of the prostate or, more importantly, of a prostate cancer's aggressive tendencies. Worse still, the treatment is very often more harmful than the disease. Treatment can include major surgery, radiotherapy, castration, chemotherapy and hormone treatment. Many men will have a focus of cancer within the prostate that does not progress and cause problems. Currently there is no test to distinguish which are likely to cause problems and which are not.

Michael Wilkes and Gavin Yamey, Editor and Deputy editor of the *Western Medical Journal*, based in California, reported their experiences in the *British Medical Journal (BMJ)*.[19] They had written an article in the *San Francisco Chronicle* in response to a news item that a manager of a baseball team had had surgery for prostate cancer diagnosed 'after a routine blood test'. They had pointed out that the US Preventive Services Taskforce did not recommend screening for prostate cancer, and explained why. They received a large number of abusive letters and emails prompted by prostate cancer charities, and there were calls to dismiss them from their posts as 'incompetent impostors'. The authors said that they had stepped on the toes of a powerful pro-screening lobby that stands to make money from encouraging men to be tested. On the other hand much of the righteous indignation was probably genuine. The general public (and many health professionals) have a simplistic view of cancer screening. This view is that 'cancer begins as a small, localised tumour which grows and eventually spreads. If the cancer can be detected and removed at an early stage before there has been any spread, it can be cured'. Therefore, in this simplistic view, detection of early cancers will save lives. In the case of prostate cancer screening, raised PSA levels do not correlate well with whether there is a cancer present that requires treatment.

Screening for testicular cancer

Testicular tumours are the most common cancers in young males between the ages of 20 and 40 years, affecting two to ten males per 100 000 per year. Ninety-two per cent are malignant, and overall they account for 1–2% of all male malignancies. Despite a slow increase in observed incidence, there has been a dramatic improvement in survival as a result of new treatments. Unlike most other cancers, this disease is generally found in young men.[20] There is a high probability (more than 50%) that a solid swelling affecting the body of the testis represents a cancer. If the swelling is not obviously solid there is a low probability of it being due to cancer, particularly in men over the age of 55 years, and you should consider arranging an ultrasound investigation before referral.

    The patient usually finds the lump, either by chance or by self-examination. Some are discovered by routine physical examination. No studies seem to have been done to find out how effective testicular self-examination or clinical testicular examination would be in reducing mortality from testicular cancer. Incomplete or non-descent of the testis is a predisposing factor for testicular tumours, increasing the risk 30-fold. Although there has been no appreciable change in how advanced the cancer is at diagnosis, advances in treatment have been associated with a 60% decrease in mortality.

Most tumours are either seminomas or teratomas. Seminomas have a good prognosis. They are radio-sensitive, there is a 90% cure rate for the early stage I and stage II disease, it remains localised for long periods before spreading to lymph nodes and bloodstream spread occurs late. Teratomas are less common than seminomas but offer a worse prognosis. With no trophoblastic element, there is a 90% cure rate for stage I disease but 60% present with stage II–IV disease and spread by the bloodstream occurs early. Overall, for all malignant tumours the five-year survival rate is about 50% if treated with orchidectomy and radiotherapy or chemotherapy.

    Most testicular cancer is so curable and there are so few cases that it would be virtually impossible to document a decrease in mortality associated with screening. Despite this, self-examination is often vigorously promoted.

Further reading on screening

You will find all of these books interesting and informative while you learn more about the difficulties inherent in screening.

Gigerenzer G (2003) *Reckoning with Risk.* Penguin Books, London.

Clarke R and Croft P (1998) *Critical Reading for the Reflective Practitioner.* Butterworth-Heinemann, Oxford.

Jordan K, Ong BN and Croft P (1998) *Mastering Statistics: a guide for health service professionals and researchers.* Stanley-Thornes, Cheltenham.

References

1 Clarke R and Croft P (1998) *Critical Reading for the Reflective Practitioner.* Butterworth-Heinemann, Oxford.

2 Jordan K, Ong BN and Croft P (1998) *Mastering Statistics: a guide for health service professionals and researchers.* Stanley-Thornes, Cheltenham.

3 Muir Gray JA (1994) Testing a test. *Bandolier* **5**: 1. http://ebandolier.com.

4 Olsen O and Gøtzsche PC (2001) Cochrane review on screening for breast cancer with mammography. *Lancet* **358**: 1340–42.

5 Nystrom I, Andersson I, Bjurstam N *et al* (2002) Long-term effects of mammography screening: updated overview of the Swedish randomised trails. *Lancet* **359**: 909–19.

6 Humphrey LL, Helfand M, Benjamin KS *et al.* (2002) Breast cancer screening: a summary of the evidence for the US Preventive Services Task Force. *Annals of Internal Medicine* **137**: 347–60.

7 Harvey J, Webb A and Mallinson H (2000) *Chlamydia trachomatis* screening in young people in Merseyside. *British Journal of Family Planning and Reproductive Health Care* **26** (4): 199–201.

8 Basarab A, Browning D, Lanham S and O'Connell S (2002) Pilot study to assess the presence of *Chlamydia trachomatis* in urine from 18–30 year-old males using EIA/IF and PCR. *British Journal of Family Planning and Reproductive Health Care* **28** (1): 36–7.

9 Foord-Kelcey G (ed) (2002) *Guidelines, Vol. 18.* Medendium Group Publishing Ltd, Berhampstead.

10 Scottish Intercollegiate Guideline Network (SIGN) (2000) *Management of Genital* Chlamydia trachomatis *Infection.* SIGN, Edinburgh.

11 Wakley G and Chambers R (2002). *Sexual Health Matters in Primary Care.* Radcliffe Medical Press, Oxford.

12 Wilkinson C and Massil H (2000) An interface of *Chlamydia* testing by community family planning clinics and referral to hospital genitourinary clinics. *British Journal of Family Planning and Reproductive Health Care* **26** (4): 206–9.

13 Gleave T (2001) Management of *Chlamydia trachomatis* in a women's hospital: a review of current practice. *Journal of Family Planning and Reproductive Health Care* **27** (3): 161–2.

14 Department of Health (2001) *The National Strategy for Sexual Health and HIV.* Department of Health, London. Also on www.doh.gov.uk/nshs.

15 Newell ML, Thorne C, Pembrey L *et al.* (1999) Antenatal screening for hepatitis B infection and syphilis in the UK. *British Journal of Obstetrics and Gynaecology* **106** (1): 66–71.

16 Austoker J, Davey C and Jansen C (1997) *Improving the Quality of the Written Information Sent to Women about Cervical Screening.* NHSCSP Publications, Sheffield.

17 Department of Health (1999) *Bulletin on Cervical Screening Programme: England 1998–9.* Department of Health, London. Also available on www.doh.gov.uk/public/sb9932.htm.

18 Chambers R, Wakley G and Iqbal Z (2001) *Cardiovascular Disease Matters in Primary Care.* Radcliffe Medical Press, Oxford.

19 Yamey G and Wilkes M (2002) The PSA storm. *British Medical Journal* **324**: 431.

20 Ries LA, Kosary CL, Hankey BF *et al.* (eds) (1998) *SEER Cancer Statistics Review 1973–1995.* National Cancer Institute, Bethesda.

6

Using contraception

Access and availability arrangements

Although the public (adult) perception is that contraception is widely and easily   **1**
available, it does not seem like that for young people. They often have considerable difficulty finding out how to obtain contraception. Even if they know
where to get it, they may not be able to get there, or feel afraid of attending.

It is a big step for someone to decide that they are sexually active and in need   **2**
of contraception. Research shows that one-fifth of teenage girls did not use
contraception the first time they had sexual intercourse. Girls tend to believe
that they should fit in with what men want in the way of a feminine image –
believing that 'romance' and 'being in love' are important. Boys adopt a
competitive masculine style and believe that risk taking is part of 'being a man'.
They may perceive that being ready and willing for sex is part of that male
persona – getting 'notches on their gun'.
   Women's experience of sexuality does not fit into the two extremes of a
whore with sexual feelings or a pure maiden with no sexual feelings at all.
Bombarded with images, clichés and media distortions, it is hardly surprising
that young people are confused.
   Traditional roles for women are similarly confused, particularly by the media
representations of how they should behave. Women see their bodies, particularly young attractive bodies, exploited as a commodity to sell almost every-
thing. Women's bodies are presented as objects that must conform to criteria of
being thin, spotless and dressed in designer garments. Young men cannot live
up to their idols of pop stars, TV characters or footballers. Teenagers feel that
they cannot achieve this ideal as many are naturally plump, with acne and on a
low income, unable to purchase fashionable clothes. No place here either for
the teenager in the wheelchair, or one with a hearing aid.

Places to obtain contraception include: **1**

- young people's clinics
- Family Planning (FP) clinics
- general practice surgeries

- shops and vending machines for condoms
- pharmacies for emergency contraceptive pills, condoms and spermicides as well as dispensing prescribed contraceptives
- NHS Direct may supply emergency contraception in some areas, as may a few accident and emergency centres.

Clinics are often listed in the *Yellow Pages* and other telephone directories under 'clinics', but unless people ring to find out it is often not clear whether there is a young people's clinic, or a FP clinic, at that site. It takes some courage to find out if there is contraceptive advice available, especially if the telephone is answered by a general receptionist or by the local district nurse! The clinic might just provide a baby clinic and chiropody and there is only sometimes an indication of what services are available. In some areas, times of opening are also listed. Leaflets about clinics are sometimes available for collection from youth clubs and other venues where young people meet.

Brook clinics that cater specifically for young people are available in many big cities. Other clinics providing contraception may be known by locally specific names.

Nationally you can find out where most clinics are situated from:

http://www.fpa.org.uk
http://www.brook.org.uk
http://lovelife.uk.com
http://ruthinking.co.uk – this site also has a free phone helpline –
0800 28 29 30, 7 a.m. to midnight – and is very 'teenage friendly'.

Oral contraceptives like the Pill are usually available from general practices and from all FP, sexual health and young people's clinics. People wanting to start the Pill usually have to see either a doctor or a nurse with special qualifications, but can often see a nurse with basic contraceptive training for follow-up checks.

Clinics, and some general practices, supply condoms, injectable hormonal contraceptives, IUD devices and contraceptive implants. Sometimes these services, especially intrauterine (IUD) devices and implants, are only available in particular clinics or surgeries and people have to go to other premises to get them. Generally the larger the general practice, the more likely it is that there will be health professionals with the expertise to supply these methods – but some small practices may also have an enthusiast! Condoms are only available from general practices in some areas with special funding.

It is not well known that patients can register with any general practice for contraceptive services separately from general medical services. This should be made clear at all of those general practices that are prepared to make provision for patients to be registered for contraceptive services only. The reception staff need to know and notices explaining the policy should be visible.

Think about how you can:

- help to make sure services are welcoming
- make provision for individuals – especially young people – to be seen quickly and at a time they can attend
- ensure that confidentiality is clearly advertised
- counter the myths about contraception, the risks of getting pregnant and that babies give you love back
- help people to be assertive with each other and only to have sex when they want to
- find out what people need, when and how
- use language that people understand
- ensure that the standards of provision and expertise are good enough.

Much of the advice and routine management of contraceptive care in healthy patients can be undertaken by properly qualified and experienced practice nurses, school nurses, midwives and health visitors.

The *Effective Health Care Bulletin* article on preventing and reducing the adverse effects of unintended teenage pregnancies[1] gives several useful messages for those providing contraceptive and reproductive healthcare to teenagers:

- *'School-based sex education can be effective in reducing teenage pregnancy, especially when linked to contraceptive services'*. So consider how you can link with local schools and school nurses.
- *'Contraceptives are highly cost-effective and can result in significant savings when used properly'*. Make sure that you have recent and accurate information yourself and that you have the skills and resources to help young people learn how to use contraception effectively.
- *'Increasing the availability of contraceptive clinic services for young people is associated with reduced pregnancy rates'*. Know about and publicise the availability of special teenage clinics. Encourage the development of youth-orientated clinics in places accessible to teenagers and open at times they can attend.
- *'Contraceptive services should be based on an assessment of local needs and ensure accessibility and confidentiality'*. Teenagers who live in rural communities, or are disadvantaged by disability, find it particularly difficult to access confidential contraceptive services.

Consultations with young people

- Discuss the guidelines on confidentiality with all young people.
- Always give the option of being seen alone.

- Follow up more frequently initially to build trust and confidence.
- Pelvic examination should only be considered if pathology is expected.
- Know the local procedures for child protection in case you learn that a young person is at risk of suffering or significant harm.
- Know and follow the 'Fraser guidelines' for advice and prescription for the under-16 year old (see below).[2]

Guidelines for advice and treatment for young people

There is no lower age limit for young people to be seen in general practices or clinics. The younger the person, the more concern there is that the person may be subject to coercion or abuse, and the more care is needed to establish whether the young person is competent, under the Fraser guidelines, to understand the implications of sexual activity and contraception.

The Fraser guidelines (previously often known as the Gillick guidelines)[2] were drawn up after a Law Lords' decision in 1985. Lord Fraser gave their judgement that a doctor can give contraceptive advice or treatment to a person under 16 years old without parental consent, providing that the doctor is satisfied that:

- the young person will understand the advice
- the young person cannot be persuaded to tell their parents or allow the doctor to tell them that they are seeking contraceptive advice
- the young person is likely to begin or continue having unprotected sex with or without contraceptive treatment
- the young person's physical or mental health is likely to suffer unless they receive contraceptive advice or treatment
- it is in the young person's best interest to be given contraceptive advice or treatment.

Fears about a potential lack of confidentiality prevent many people attending their own doctor or practice nurse about sexual health matters. Even at clinics away from their home area, people fear that their details will be passed on without their consent. Practices and clinics need to consider how to record information and how to control who has access to that information. Teenagers often believe that their details will be divulged to parents or other adults who they fear will be critical. Clear messages about confidentiality help to allay the anxieties.

You may be asked to keep what you are told completely confidential. You should always qualify any assurance you give about confidentiality with a caveat about the need to break confidentiality if the adolescent or other person is at serious risk of harm.

The Royal College of General Practitioners/Brook training kit enables general practices to think through four scenarios illustrating difficult situations where confidentiality issues arise.[3] Practice teams can discuss and agree their policies on confidentiality for young teenagers. The training kit encourages practices to advertise their policy clearly in the practice leaflet, advising teenagers that they can go for contraceptive help to any other practice, with contact details of doctors nearby who are happy to see them.

This kit would be a useful way of exploring the issues for anyone who is not sure how they might proceed in any given situation.

Outreach and innovative services[4]

Family planning-trained nurses in North Staffordshire and elsewhere are extending their roles by operating a 'clinic-in-a-box'. They go to settings where other facilities for young people are being provided (coffee, snooker, table tennis etc.). They take supplies of condoms, emergency and oral contraception, leaflets and other information and are available to listen and give advice. They can prescribe under group directives. The young people feel that they are 'on their own ground' and are often much more forthcoming that in more traditional 'medical' settings. This provision is particularly useful to engage the attention of young men.

The End House project in Durham was set up in response to findings from local research on young people's needs. A three-storey building with a shop front houses various support services for young people, and includes contraceptive clinic provision.

The Park House project in north Tyneside provides a venue used solely by young people wanting to access sexual health services. The young people gain access via an intercom system so that every person is individually welcomed into the building. The building provides a confidential but welcoming and user-friendly service. It also provides 'C-cards' so that young people can obtain free condoms from a variety of other outlets.

The Burnham young adult drop-in clinic in Somerset provides a comprehensive sexual health service as well as more general health services for young people. A separate entrance, as well as a separate record and filing system, have provided an obviously confidential service.

'The Van' in Wakefield parks in the evening in areas that have been agreed with young people in advance. Youth workers staff the van and are able to issue condoms and give advice about any sort of health or social problem. They can direct young people to one of the seven young people's clinics in the area for further contraceptive advice or supplies.

3

In some areas outreach workers provide condoms and advice to sex workers. This reduces infection as well as pregnancy.

Clinics in schools have been set up in various parts of the UK. In rural areas, a clinic at lunchtime can be the only way to access confidential help for young people who live in country areas with no public transport. It is even more difficult to access help for your sexual needs if you have to ask a parent or other adult for a lift to the nearest doctor or clinic!

Think about how you might go about increasing the availability of good contraceptive advice to those who need it. Find out what the consumers of contraceptive advice would like (see Chapter 3). Consider making the provision as flexible as possible. Some clinics see anyone who walks in; other busier clinics may have to ask if the patient can wait to be fitted in after patients with appointments have been seen. Think about the following when making arrangements and ask young people what they prefer:

- People who book into a *general surgery session* do not have to state the reason for attending, either to the receptionist, or tacitly to the other patients in the waiting area, or to people at work or at home who might want to know where they are going. The disadvantage is that lack of time or expertise may prevent adequate discussion if contraceptive or sexual health needs are complex.
- People who book into a *designated clinic* may be better able to state to the world that they are sexually active. They expect to have more specialised attention and expertise in a clinic. It is usually possible to give more time for more complex consultations. Giving the clinic a name other than 'family planning' and carrying out some other functions (such as cervical smears or well-person checks) may make it easier to people to state that they wish to attend that clinic. Many clinics for young people have names thought up by the young people themselves and often offer other services as well as contraception and sexual health.

Cultural issues

Every individual or couple attending for advice on fertility control has a unique need. In addition to those considerations arising from the medical history, others are derived from their particular ethnic, social, family and cultural backgrounds. The background of healthcare staff can give rise to conflicts with the belief systems of the patients whose contraceptive requirements they need to meet. The first step is to understand our own beliefs and values and how they are based on our own culture and upbringing. Then we need to understand what the issues might be for others from different groups or communities. Particularly we need to guard against stereotyping others.

This is not to say that learning about other people's religious and cultural beliefs is not useful. A framework of knowledge helps to make bridges and increase understanding. For example, knowing that some religions believe that life begins at fertilisation and not after implantation helps you to explore someone's beliefs before spending unproductive time discussing an unacceptable method. Similarly, knowing a little about religious festivals or observances helps with understanding a woman's reluctance to consider a contraceptive method that might cause bleeding at a time that is unacceptable. You might want to make a start by reading a book[5] or gather information from the patients you see. It may seem frustrating to someone from a 'liberated Western culture' that a woman must return home to discuss what she is to do about contraception with her husband, or with her mother-in-law. Always be ready to admit your ignorance and ask for explanations. Understanding the religious or cultural aspects will help the healthcare worker to accept behaviour or beliefs, and help the individual to trust the healthcare worker as respecting their particular needs. The patient is then more likely to trust other advice as being in their best interest rather than as a solution imposed on them from an alien set of values. Always find out what would be useful for that individual and do not assume that the opinions of one person from a culture or religion tell you what another person from that culture or religion will need.

Many religions support procreation and disapprove of contraception, but personal needs and beliefs may be quite different. Many people decide for themselves how much notice they take of cultural or religious pronouncements, but may have guilt and difficulties because of ambivalent feelings. Young women with little ambition or poor education may also use no contraception or use it erratically because of feelings of powerlessness, or that the only thing that they can do well, or be valued for, is to have babies. In every consultation, establish what the beliefs are for the woman or for the couple, so that the choice of method will be suitable for them at that time.

Cultural influences also affect how people are viewed as sexual beings. A woman over 40 years of age may find it uncomfortable attending the same clinic session as groups of teenagers, who, she feels, look at her in undisguised amazement. She may have preferred to attend a different session where more of her age group are likely to be present, but have been directed to this one because her need for contraception is urgent. She needs consideration of her special needs in just the same way as a lone teenager requiring emergency contraception who is fitted into a well-person clinic dealing mainly with menopausal women.

Culture may also affect the way in which people with disabilities are viewed. People with any disability are often regarded as not having any sexual needs and therefore not in need of contraception. Sexual health provision for people with visual or auditory handicaps is often poor. Having to ask where the family planning clinic is because you cannot see the notice, or being unable to hear your name called when you have been waiting to be seen, can be very off-putting. Coping with healthcare staff who do not know how best to help you is another hurdle! Physical handicaps may prevent access to buildings with steps or on upper floors without lifts. Information is rarely available in large print, Braille or on tape. Unless people with disabilities can find able-bodied companions to help them, they are often unable to obtain or use contraception.

Cultural or religious considerations may also affect whether people feel that they can access particular services. If a clinic is situated in an area perceived as rough, or looks run down and vandalised, it may not be used by people who find this threatening or unacceptable. Just as off-putting are smart new premises in leafy suburbs to the disadvantaged in society, who perceive such provision as being prejudiced against them. So a variety of provision is necessary to cater for all perceptions. What is essential is the welcome afforded – the word soon gets around if the reception staff and health professionals are non-judgemental and helpful.

Delivering the messages about contraception

Peer education is heralded as a key influence and positive force in many current schemes to reduce teenage pregnancy. The extent of regretted first intercourse highlights the significant negative pressures that many youngsters are under from their peers to embark on sexual activity. Rates of reported coercion increase with younger age at first intercourse.

3

Television is thought to help young people define cultural norms and influence their perceptions of the real world and acceptable social behaviour. Television, radio, newspapers and magazines are all popular media for delivering preventive health messages and are often seen as appropriate ways to engage young people.

The influence of the media and of advertising has been blamed as one of the contributory factors in encouraging teenagers to become sexually active at an earlier age.

A national omnibus survey of parents and teens conducted in 1999 explored parents' views about 'who or what influences your teen child or children most, besides their boyfriend or girlfriend, when it comes to decisions about sex'.[6] Eleven per cent thought that 'television, movies and musicians' exerted the most influence on their teenage offspring, compared to 55% who thought that parents or guardians had most influence; 14% believed that peers were most influential and 13% considered religion to carry most weight. When young people themselves were asked the same question, 8% thought that 'television, movies and musicians' had most influence on their decisions about sex, as opposed to parents or guardians (38%), peers (25%) and religion (14%). The majority of parents and teenagers considered that teachers had little influence on teenagers' decision making about sex, with 0.3% of parents and 2% of teenagers thinking that teachers were the most important figures in young people's lives in influencing their decisions about sex.

The power of the media to influence teenagers' behaviour has been demonstrated by health promotion campaigns. Both the intensity and duration over which the messages are delivered appear to be important. The mass media may be a particularly appropriate medium for relaying health promotion messages. The messages are regarded as more credible when relayed by the mass media as opposed to school programmes because high-risk youngsters are greatly exposed to and interested in the media – a British Audience Research Bureau report showed that 4–15 year olds watched an average 19 hours of television per week and 16–24 year olds watched 20 hours of television per week.[6]

Radio can reach other groups of people who may listen 'on the move' rather than watching television at home.

Teen idols can influence other teenagers to follow their example to provide encouragement to girls and young women who find themselves under pressure from boyfriends to give in to sexual demands. In America, self-declared teenage celibates are known as 'pledge keepers'.

The Internet is generally seen as a useful resource that has the potential to supply information about health to aid understanding and empower that person in any medical consultation. This bodes well for the young person seeking information about sexuality or contraception, so long as the information is accurate and reliable. Sexual health promotion via the Internet may be more open to abuse than other health topics. Children may access sexual health sites where explicit material is unsuitable, or be exploited by pornographers or extremists. Any site that uses the word 'sex' in its title is likely to be subject to parental or provider controls. Health Development Agency principles are intended to safeguard the use of the Internet for sexual health promotion:

- All communications should be accompanied by a detailed brief explaining what public health outcomes and health impact are intended.
- Recognise the diversity of sexual attitudes and sexual lifestyles and avoid being judgemental.
- Promote mutual self-respect, and the benefits to well-being from caring and emotionally fulfilling relationships.
- Messages should be accurate, clear and honest where there is uncertainty about the evidence.
- The target audience should be carefully defined.
- The language should be justified by its purpose and intended outcome.
- All materials should be pre-tested and modified in response to research findings before being released.

Magazines were judged to be an important source of information in a study seeking to understand the factors that influence young people in their sexual behaviour and their attitudes towards pregnancy. Problem pages were regarded as being particularly useful.[6]

Myths

Some of the misunderstandings or misinterpretations that can affect people's sexual lives are discussed below. Some of them are ideas prevalent amongst young people (and some older people too); others are due to out-of-date medical knowledge or misunderstandings of the way in which fertility or fertility control works.

The World Health Organization dispelled the myth that sex education has caused unwanted pregnancies and earlier sexual activity. It examined 19 studies and concluded that sex and HIV/AIDS education does not promote earlier or increased sexual activity in young people. In fact, such education leads to a greater uptake of safer sexual practices. In the UK, school sex education is still treated warily and depends very much on the attitudes of the governors and staff in individual schools. Numerous surveys of young people have concluded that they have too little information and often too late. Fifteen years ago pregnancy rates across Europe were very similar. Studies by the Guttmacher Institute of 32 developed countries have shown that teenage pregnancy rates have fallen, particularly in the Netherlands, Sweden and Denmark. These countries have good sex education programmes and contraceptive services for young people and the discussion of sexual activity is much more open than in the UK. They have much lower teenage pregnancy rates than the UK, and their teenagers delay sexual activity to a later age than in the UK. The UK has the highest teenage pregnancy rates in Western Europe.[6]

Common myths about sexual activity in the UK

Many teenagers worry if they are still virgins at 15, 16 or 17 years old. They believe that nearly everyone else is sexually active, except them. In the National Survey of Sexual Attitudes and Lifestyles, 19% of female teenagers and 28% of males currently aged 16–19 years old reported that they had their first sexual intercourse before the age of 16 years.[6] That means over 80% of girls and nearly three-quarters of boys had *not* had sexual intercourse before the age of 16 years. Unfortunately, if adults tell them this they do not believe it — only if it comes from their own peer group. With acute perception, they see that adults would like them not to be sexually active and think that this information is part of the plot to control their sexuality. To admit to being a virgin, or even to wanting to stay one, appears to be unacceptable and not conforming to the norms of their peer group. So people pretend and lie about their experiences, even to the point of taking contraceptives that they do not need.

Other ideas that cause difficulties — not just in the teenage years — are that all physical contact must lead to sex, that sex is penetration, that a man is always ready to have sex and that a man should not express emotions such as tenderness. These ideas lead to the mentality that sexual activity is about 'getting notches on your gun' or having sex with as many different partners as possible.

There is still pressure on young men to initiate sex, to believe that it is the performance that counts, not the person or how well you get on together. Especially when both are inexperienced, it is no wonder that so many young teenagers are disappointed by their early sexual encounters. They are unaware that it takes time and practice to produce a good performance at any skill, including sexual intercourse.

Many of the Victorian ideas about the differences between males and females still exist and are often perpetuated in magazines. It is still possible to read articles about 'how to satisfy your man' and others implying that women do not enjoy sex as much as men. It is suggested that men prefer inhibited women, or that they feel threatened by the woman taking the lead. Of course, some do, but others will find it more arousing — generalisations about people's sexuality are not useful for individual couples. Teenage girls worry about what a boy will think of them if they prepare for sexual activity by going on the Pill or carrying condoms. Will he think she is too forward, not a 'nice' girl or ready to have sex with just anyone? Will she get a reputation of being too 'easy'?

More dangerously, the myth that women say 'no' when they mean 'yes' is still held by a small minority of men. These attitudes can lead to date rape, or at least to coercive sexual intercourse.

The feelings that exciting sex involves risk, or that sex should always be natural and spontaneous, often result in the lack of use of contraception. If you believe that sexual intercourse should follow being swept off your feet in a turmoil of passion, you can hardly plan contraception in advance! Disappointment often follows, and what many teenagers attending for emergency contraception say about their sexual experience is that they felt let down or cheated by the lack of feeling.

The attitude that sex is not talked about, or if it is, only by innuendo and embarrassed laughter is taking a long time to disappear from the UK. The view that, 'if you don't mention sex, teenagers will not be interested in it', has been disproved over and over again. If you have no practice at talking about sexual activity at home in an open and matter-of-fact way, you are more likely to find it difficult to negotiate the use of a condom when starting sexual intercourse with a new partner. If you cannot talk about sex, how will you know when to start on contraception, or where to obtain it from? Of course, prurient interest in the details of young people's sexual activity is almost as off putting — sexual activity is private and the relationship precious. However, a parent or guardian not asking if contraception is needed or whether it has been considered is likely to lead to absence of contraception and the presence of unwanted pregnancy instead.

Common myths held and why they are untrue

- *You can't get pregnant*:
  - *if it's your first time.* Untrue — it only takes a few seconds for the sperm to reach the egg.
  - *if you do it twice in a row, or one day after another, or the second time, you don't need a condom because there are no sperm left.* Every ejaculate contains over 300 million sperm.
  - *if you are not doing it often.* You are *less* likely to become pregnant, but still running a risk.
  - *if you don't have an orgasm.* Orgasm is not necessary to draw the sperm into the uterus — they swim quite well without!
  - *because he's been doing it for ages and not got anyone pregnant yet.* Intercourse with someone else is no guarantee for this relationship.
  - *if he presses in the groin before ejaculating to prevent the sperm from getting out.* The sperm are already in the seminal vesicles in the prostate gland long before orgasm is imminent.
  - *if you have sex standing up, or if you have a bath after sex.* It only takes a few seconds for the sperm to reach the egg, even uphill.
- *Withdrawal is useless.* It is better than nothing, but back it up with emergency contraception.
- *It is easy to work out when you will be fertile by counting 14 days from the first day of your last period.* Ovulation occurs about 14 days before the next period. Few women have exactly regular 28-day cycles and illness or other events, including use of emergency contraception, may delay the next period. Sperm live for up to seven days in the genital tract but the egg can only be fertilised up to about 12 hours after release.
- *You cannot be given contraception until you are 16 years old.* Untrue, and being under 16 years old is no protection against becoming pregnant.
- *Every tenth condom has a hole in it.* Condoms with a CE mark (which replaces the kite mark) are safe and very thoroughly tested.
- *If you use two condoms it will be safer than one.* Condoms may be more likely to tear because of friction.
- *'I can't fit into a condom.'* Condoms stretch 15 feet! If it doesn't fit, it is probably not put on correctly.

2

- *It's better if you use Vaseline as a lubricant.* Grease or oil-based lubricants weaken condoms.
- *'I'm too young to get you pregnant.'* If he can be sexually active he may be capable of getting someone pregnant.
- *'I can't get pregnant when I'm just off my period.'* It is less likely but tests have shown that some people can produce an egg that early in the menstrual cycle.
- *'It's safe as long as I urinate before and after sex.'* Urine doesn't kill sperm and will not wash sperm away safely.

Many other false ideas about contraception abound. It is common for people to believe that contraception is dangerous to health, without comparing it to the risks of pregnancy, which are much higher.

Always ask about worries that people have and treat them sympathetically. Don't laugh or treat the idea with scorn. Many of the myths come from accepting what someone else has said, or from too little information. Acknowledge the sense behind the idea, e.g. saying 'I can see how you might think that', so that people can bring up other false ideas. Then explain tactfully why the information they have is wrong.

Condoms and barrier methods

General information

The failure rate for condoms is around 3% per year (that is, three in a hundred people who use condoms for a year would get pregnant) but varies according to how carefully they are used.

Many shapes and colours of condoms are available, but remember no matter how much fun they are they have a job to do and need to be used properly. Make sure that the condom packet has a CE mark on it to ensure that it reaches very high standards of quality control. Modern condoms are thinner and are quick and easy to use.

Lots of women, like lots of men, carry condoms with them, not because they are easy for sex but because they want to protect themselves. Condoms may be bought in many places, including chemists, garages, supermarkets, some toilets and they are free from FP clinics. General practices in some areas are able to supply them free also.

Some simple facts

- Always put the condom on before the penis touches the other person's genitals.

- Never put them on or touch them with long, jagged nails or sharp jewellery as they can tear.
- Don't get perfume or deodorants near them.
- You can use lubricants that do *not* have perfume, oil or grease in them (such as KY jelly, Sensilube or a spermicide cream or jelly).
- Don't believe the myth that condoms burst easily. They will stretch to 15 feet and can hold up to 16 pints of water.
- After ejaculation, hold the end of the condom onto the penis and withdraw.
- A condom can slip off. If it does, advise people to seek emergency contraception.
- After use, wrap them in paper and put them in a bin.

Advisors and providers of condoms need to be comfortable discussing how a condom should be used, and in suggesting ways in which it can be incorporated into love play (the woman putting the condom on the man can be very arousing). Suggest that the man practises putting a condom on his erect penis before he will need to in the heat of the moment — when it may be difficult to remember what to do. A woman can practise on a suitably shaped substitute!

Suggest that a condom is always carried in a pocket or wallet. Girls can put one in a purse or inside their bra before they go out to a party — they often do not have pockets.

Negotiating the use of a condom can be quite tricky. If you suggest using a condom without tact, the other person may *hear* that you think they are dirty or have slept around. It is better to use language that includes both of the couple like 'If we use a condom, it stops either of us catching any germs from the other one' or 'To show we both care for each other we should use a condom'.

Using a suitable lubricant can improve sensitivity and prevent breakage. Lubricants are often sold on the same counter as condoms in chemists and supermarkets. A better range is available by mail order, from Anne Summers shops and from sex shops. Sex is fun after all!

People often prefer to use condoms because they can buy them without having to see a health professional. This increases their sense of confidentiality, but may mean that they have to travel outside the area in which they live to buy them, or check that no one they know is around before making their purchase.

Choice of condoms

Female condoms (Femidom) need to be used carefully to avoid positioning the penis so that it is not covered. They are rather expensive but can be bought over the counter with no need for medical intervention. They are disliked by some because of the 'plastic mac' feel and are noisy in use.

Male condoms are sold in many different shapes and sizes. They also come in various colours or with added knobs or ribbing. The variety adds to the fun. Collect a selection of different ones so that you can show people what they look like — and perhaps more important, how they feel. Modern condoms have improved dramatically and can feel very silky and sensuous. The size varies as well. A condom should fit snugly without being tight, and have room at the tip for the ejaculate. Some are straight-sided, others shaped. If the condom slips off it may be too small (so it does not roll down properly), too wide (so it does not grip the base of the shaft) or have too small a space at the end (the ejaculate pushes it off the snug fit).

Extra strong condoms are available for anal sex and should always be used with lubricant.

Other barrier methods

Failure rates for diaphragms and caps depend very much on the user for both the accuracy of the fit and to actually use it for every act of intercourse. Failure rates are 5% per year with perfect use but as high as 21% per year with typical use. **2**

Having a diaphragm or cap fitted involves a vaginal examination and this may deter some people. The diaphragm or cap must always be used together with a spermicide. Good teaching and practice are essential to ensure that the device and pool of spermicide cover the cervix.

Most caps or diaphragms are fitted and supplied by clinics. A disposable cap can be bought from chemists, but a fitting set has to be bought and taken to a clinic to ensure the correct size is purchased.

The degree of organisation and forward planning required for reliable use makes the diaphragm a more suitable choice for those in stable, long-term relationships. It also requires access to (preferably private) washing facilities and convenient storage.

Dental dams can be used to prevent infection during oral sex. One side need to be marked so that if it falls off, it can be replaced in the original position. A condom split along one side can be used in the same way.

Barrier methods and disability

Putting in a diaphragm or cap made slippery with spermicide can be a challenge to fully able-bodied women, let alone when physical disability impairs mobility or dexterity. Involving the partner can be an advantage, as can shared responsibility for putting on a condom. Four handicapped hands can substitute for two **3** fully functional ones. Remember that people with learning disabilities tend to take teaching very literally, so be very clear about where the diaphragm or condom is to be fitted. Using a model may be confusing and lead to incorrect use. Advice about emergency contraception should always accompany instruction about barrier methods.

Spermicides

Nonoxinol-9 has been widely used in spermicides for contraception over the **3** past 50 years. In the 1970s and 1980s, laboratory tests showed it could destroy the micro-organisms responsible for HIV, gonorrhoea and chlamydia. The initial excitement of this discovery spawned a whole series of clinical investigations of nonoxinol-9's protective effect against transmission of STIs. Much of this work was necessarily in very high-risk groups like sex workers, in developing countries with high rates of HIV/AIDS. The results were disappointing, suggesting that the spermicide might actually increase the risk of HIV transmission in these groups, perhaps by causing mucosal irritation and ulceration.

Since then condom manufacturers have been discontinuing making condoms lubricated with nonoxinol-9. Used infrequently the spermicide does not appear to cause damage to the vaginal walls, but it is not now recommended for people who have frequent sexual intercourse.

Research on new spermicides is continuing and looks hopeful, but is not at the commercial stage yet.

Drugs and prostitution

Drugs lower inhibitions. Many young people report that they had unprotected **3** intercourse while under the influence of alcohol or cannabis. Emergency contraception and infection screening should follow exposure. Everyone needs greater awareness of the risks.

People with greater self-esteem and self-assertiveness can say 'No' to too much alcohol, illegal drugs *and* unwanted intercourse.

One study of drug injectors in England estimated that 7–10% had accepted money or drugs for sex. The majority of professional prostitutes of either sex know the risks, and the levels of HIV infection among female prostitutes are low. In Glasgow, all of the female prostitutes who were found to be HIV-positive (2.3%) were also drug injectors. Drug users or professional sex workers should take appropriate precautions, e.g. using stronger condoms.

Male prostitutes are often at a disadvantage. They are usually paid after the transaction, and the client usually makes the decision about condoms. Female prostitutes are often adept at applying condoms in an exciting way, and either refuse a client or charge much higher fees for sex without a condom as a deterrent. Those most at risk are drug users or the homeless who sell sex for drugs, food or shelter.[7]

Condoms and starting relationships

If you believe that sexuality is only acceptable if you are male, then women believe that if they carry condoms they will be branded as sluts.[1] Women often know about safe sex and intend to use condoms, but find themselves unable to be assertive enough within the context of a sexual relationship. They feel that they should be passive and undemanding and that the man should take the lead.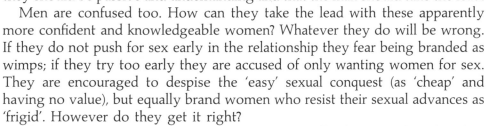

Men are confused too. How can they take the lead with these apparently more confident and knowledgeable women? Whatever they do will be wrong. If they do not push for sex early in the relationship they fear being branded as wimps; if they try too early they are accused of only wanting women for sex. They are encouraged to despise the 'easy' sexual conquest (as 'cheap' and having no value), but equally brand women who resist their sexual advances as 'frigid'. However do they get it right?

Check too that using a barrier method will not offend against the cultural or religious values held by either of the couple. Some religions and cultures hold that barriers are unnatural or are proscribed. Don't make assumptions if you note that someone is of a particular culture or religion. Find out exactly how they understand any restrictions placed on them.[6]

Contraceptive methods

Choice of method

No one method will suit everyone, and people will choose different methods at **1** different stages of their lives. No ideal method exists, and all methods fail — some more often than others. If it is important to avoid pregnancy then a more reliable method should be chosen. You might use a good up-to-date reference manual such as the FPA's *Contraceptive Handbook*[8] or *Contraception: your questions answered*[9] for any problems or queries.

It is important to discuss some of the less reliable but neglected methods. Too often it is assumed that people will want to use the combined oral contraception pill and condoms, or the injection and condoms, because it is what health professionals would like them to use for maximum contraceptive efficacy. Sexual activity is enjoyable, but contraception is a nuisance and will be neglected or avoided unless it is the choice made by that individual. Knowing that all possibilities have been considered, the individual is not left thinking 'There must be something better than this' or 'I'm not having sex often so I won't bother with all this stuff'.

Remember to discuss the risks of infection. Using the Pill, injection or implant may give good contraceptive protection, but little or no protection against STIs. Discuss with users how they can negotiate the use of condoms as well as using a good method of contraception.

Always discuss confidentiality issues. If young people are still living at home and do not wish to discuss their contraceptive needs with parents, they must think about how to store their contraceptives and how to remember to use them as part of deciding which method to use.

Remember too that many young people spend a lot of time away from home, staying over with friends or going out for the night. They should think about how they will remember to use any method that requires regular activity, like pill taking, and whether their contraceptives will be left in the wrong place. Think about those with no fixed abode or who live in more than one home because their parents are separated – how are they to manage? They may prefer to use a method that does not require any storage such as an injection or implant.

A young woman might choose an injection or implant together with condoms to protect her while she has a chaotic lifestyle in adolescence. She might transfer to using the combined oral contraceptive (COC) once she has settled into a long-term partnership or marriage. Between pregnancies she and her partner might want to use condoms, a diaphragm or the progestogen-only pill (POP) while breast-feeding or if another pregnancy would be welcome quite soon. Once their family desires are complete, she might want to use a really effective method like an IUD or return to an implant. The couple might decide on vasectomy if they feel she has 'done her bit' and it is his turn to take the responsibility for contraception.

Effectiveness of methods

- *Abstinence*. Effectiveness: 100% used reliably; 10–20% per year if not, i.e. the background risk of becoming pregnant if no contraceptive method is used and the couple do not abstain after all.

- *Periodic abstinence or 'natural methods'*. Failure rates are difficult to establish because of the varying application of these methods but are usually quoted to be between about 2 and 20% per year.
- *Withdrawal* (coitus interruptus). Failure rate: it is difficult to establish the reliability. Studies have mainly been done in couples in stable, long-term relationships in whom the fertility rate does not seem to be increased compared with groups using barrier methods.
- *Combined oral contraceptive pills*. Failure rate: many figures given vary from 0.1–5% per year. The FPA quotes 99% contraceptive safety with consistent use.
- *Progestogen-only contraceptive pills*. Failure rate is about 2–3% per year with consistent use.
- *Progestogen injections or implants, IUDs and sterilisation*. Failure rates are less than 1% in the first year.

Remember that emergency contraception given after unprotected intercourse has a failure rate of 5% (given within 24 hours) to 42% (given at 72 hours). It is no substitute for a regular continuing method.

Table 6.1 provides a chart, derived from WHO guidelines,[10] to enable you to check if it is safe for someone to use a particular method of contraception. If the conditions listed are present, either the method should not be used (X) or you should check a reference book or the datasheet for relative contraindications or cautions (C).

Fears and misunderstandings about hormonal contraception

A common question asked is 'Isn't hormonal contraception risky?' The simple answer to this is that the Pill or an injection is less risky than a pregnancy in any healthy young woman. The reason for taking a history is to establish the few contraindications to using oestrogen-containing pills; even in these women (e.g. with focal migraine), progestogen-only methods can often be considered.

The risks of smoking (which many adolescents do) are much higher than the risks of either being pregnant or taking contraception.

Heart attacks

Women who do not smoke and do not have any other risk factors for cardiac disease are at little, if any, extra risk of myocardial infarction if they take the Pill. The relative risk of a myocardial infarction is 20 times greater in women

Table 6.1 Contraceptive methods and pre-existing conditions[10] (X = the method should not be used; C = check a reference book or datasheet for relative contraindications or cautions)

	COC	POP	Inject	Implant	IUD	IUS	Barrier
Pregnancy	X	X	X	X	X	X	
Before any pregnancies					C	C	
Hypertension	X						
Structural heart disease with significant valve problem or a septal defect	X				C		
Bacterial endocarditis (past or at risk)					X	X	
Known high risk of thrombosis due to inherited condition or immobility	X						
Inherited hyperlipidaemia	X/C						
Migraine with focal symptoms	X						
Irregular vaginal bleeding before diagnosis of cause	X	X	X	X	X	X	
Heavy or painful menstrual loss					C		
Ovarian cysts		C					
Previous ectopic pregnancy		C			C		
Septate uterus or stenosis of cervical os					X	X	
Pelvic inflammatory disease or increased risk					X	X	
Toxic shock syndrome							C
Recurrent urinary tract infections							C
Biliary tract disease or cholestasis	C	C	C	C		C	
Liver disease current or before tests have returned to normal	X	C	C	C		C	
Porphyria	X						
Wilson's disease					X		
Liver tumours	X	C	C	C		C	
Thalassaemia					C		
Sickle cell disease (not sickle cell *trait* which can be disregarded)	C				C		
Anaemias					C		
Drug interactions (rifampicin, phenytoin, carbamazepine, barbiturates, topiramate, ritonavir, or other liver enzyme inducers)	C	C	C	C			

Key to method: COC = combined oral contraceptive; POP = progestogen-only pill; IUD = intrauterine device; IUS = intrauterine system with progestogen; Inject = progestogen injectable; Implant = implant of progestogen; Barrier = diaphragm, cap, condoms.

who smoke more than 15 cigarettes daily and use the COC pill compared to non-users who do not smoke. However, the absolute risk of heart attacks in young women is very low.

Stroke

Work from the WHO emphasises the importance of a raised blood pressure and smoking in the aetiology of stroke. Both of these increase the risk of haemorrhagic stroke but the use of COCs does not. Ischaemic stroke is related to thrombosis and is increased in COC users, but the risk increases markedly in smokers. Although haemorrhagic stroke can occur at any age (although the incidence increases with age), ischaemic stroke is extremely rare in young people, and the increased risk was reported for those over 35 years old.

Venous thromboembolism (VTE)

Venous thrombosis associated with oestrogen use may occur in higher-risk   **3** women. It needs to be explained that this is not a risk to life in itself, only if it causes part of a clot to break off and travel to another part of the body (venous thromboembolism – VTE). No one should be diagnosed as having a deep venous thrombosis in the leg on the basis of leg pain or cramp alone. If there is pain in just on one leg then COCs should be stopped (and another method used) while investigations are carried out. A woman's future healthcare and contraceptive method depends on an accurate diagnosis. Clots that occur in the menstrual loss are *not* associated with any increased risk, or associated with thrombosis in any way.

Family history, if known, may be of use in predicting the likelihood of VTE, but more than 50% of people who develop VTE have no hereditary defects of coagulation that can be detected.

The WHO Scientific Group gives the risks for VTE as:

background risk – five per 100 000 women per year
in pregnancy – 60 per 100 000 pregnancies
second-generation COCs – 15 per 100 000 women per year
third-generation COCs – 25–30 per 100 000 women per year.

The media attention in 1995 surrounding the publication of evidence showing an increased risk of VTE if using third-generation COCs caused many women to stop taking the Pill altogether and be exposed to a greater risk due to pregnancy.

Types of COCs

Second-generation COCs contain levonorgestrel or norethisterone as the progestogen; third-generation COCs contain desogestrel or gestodene as the progestogen.

It is too early to categorise the new progestogen drospirenone, but it is likely to fit into the third-generation type. Dianette, while not primarily a contraceptive as it is mainly used to treat acne and hirsutism in women, has increased risks of thrombosis. The risks and benefits of this treatment should be reviewed regularly.

Low-strength COCs contain ethinyloestradiol 20 micrograms. Standard strength COCs contain 30 or 35 micrograms of ethinyloestradiol in a fixed dose throughout *or* 30/40 micrograms phased (variable) dose.

Biphasic or triphasic COCs are more complex to take but may provide better control of the bleeding pattern in some patients. They contain pills with two levels of hormones, usually seven days at a lower level and 14 at a higher level (biphasic) or seven pills at a low level of hormones, seven pills at a higher level, then a lower level of oestrogen with a higher level of progestogen for another seven days (triphasic).

Twenty-eight day packs usually contain seven inactive pills and 21 active pills containing both oestrogen and progestogen.

A high-strength COC containing 50 micrograms of ethinyloestradiol is used mainly for patients on liver enzyme-inducing drugs.

Weight

One of the major concerns of women is weight gain. Most women compare themselves with those models they see illustrated in magazines or on television. The normal change in shape (the development of hips and fatter thighs especially) that occurs in adolescence is often misinterpreted as being 'gross' and 'fat'. **1**

Weight gain is often blamed on the Pill, and even when it can be demonstrated that no change in weight has occurred, the change in shape is too much bear. Most studies of COC show that 60% of women on the Pill do not have any significant change in weight, which varies between plus or minus a couple of kilograms. About 20–25% will gain more than that and 15–20% will lose more than that. Of course, the steady increase in weight that usually occurs with increasing age has also to be taken into account. The COC Yasmin, containing the new progesterone drospirenone, is associated with less weight gain in the early months of taking it, or even some small weight loss, compared with standard preparations. However, weight changes overall in the published **2** studies were small and weight tended to creep up in the second year of use. This formulation may be of use if the main complaint is of bloating as less fluid retention occurs. You may want it as a second-choice preparation for selected users, especially as it is more expensive than older preparations.

Counselling before starting injectable progestogens is important as most women gain some weight, usually about two kilograms in the first year. A few people seem to put on weight very rapidly. Increased appetite appears to be the main cause rather than fluid retention.

Fertility fears

There used to a fashion for having regular breaks from the COC every few years. All that happened was that people had a higher risk of pregnancy while using a less efficient method and often demonstrated this with an unplanned pregnancy. In fact the COC does much to *reduce* the risks of infertility. There is less risk of pelvic infection, fewer ectopic pregnancies, less endometriosis and less risk of functional ovarian cysts, all of which may impair future fertility by pelvic adhesions, scarring or surgical interference. So there is no rational reason to have breaks from the COC or to worry about fertility – at least not until well past the teenage years when age alone may impair fertility.

Many teenagers express fears that having the progestogen injection will make them 'sterile'. This is partly muddled thinking about the purpose of regular menstruation, and partly fears about stories they have heard about people taking a long time to become pregnant after stopping it. Absence of the menstrual cycle usually does imply inability to become pregnant – but not permanently, only until ovulation is re-established, usually about 14 days before the next menstrual period arrives. After use of progestogen injections, there may be a delay before return to full fertility. The mean time to conception in a large study of women in Thailand who discontinued progestogen injections was nine months; by two years fertility rates were normal compared with users of other methods of contraception. The return to fertility is often quicker, particularly in underweight women – so the delay in the restoration of fertility should not be relied on if pregnancy is not wanted![9]

Cancer worries

Breast cancer seems a particular worry that is often out of proportion to the actual risk. A recognised risk factor for breast cancer is a late age at the time of the first full-term pregnancy – and the pill or injection delays pregnancy very effectively. The risk of breast cancer in young women is very small (one in 500 up to the age of 35 years old), so an increase in the risk will result in very small numbers of sufferers. Current Pill users experience about a 25% increase of this very small risk, but this wanes in ex-users and is not detectable 10 years after use.

Tenderness in the breast after starting hormonal contraception is *not* a sign that the woman will develop cancer later. Increases in breast cancer, cervical cancer and the very rare liver tumours need to be balanced against the reductions in uterine and ovarian cancers that occur in people using hormonal contraception. Overall the balance is probably about equal. Currently available hormonal contraception does not appear to be associated with a net excess risk. The facts about the beneficial effects of COCs are often lost in the media-induced hysteria.

The advantages and disadvantages of COCs

Advantages of COCs include:

2

- excellent protection against pregnancy
- prevention of iron deficiency by reduction of menstruation loss
- reduction of dysmenorrhoea
- reduced risk of ovarian and uterine cancer
- protection against pelvic inflammatory disease
- less benign breast disease
- fewer functional ovarian cysts
- reduction of ectopic pregnancy risk because ovulation is inhibited
- probable reduction in endometriosis
- fewer symptomatic fibroids
- probable reduction in the risk of thyroid disease, rheumatoid arthritis, possibly also duodenal ulcers
- reduction in acne for oestrogen-dominant pills.

Disadvantages include:

- requires consistent regular action by an individual
- increased risk of VTE disease as above
- increased risk of arterial disease in users who smoke, have other risk factors and with increasing age

- increases in blood pressure
- possible increase in risk of breast cancer being diagnosed while on COC and for up to 10 years afterwards (less risk of an advanced cancer being diagnosed)
- possible risk of being a co-factor for the development of cervical cancer
- possible increase in the (very rare) risk of liver tumours
- possible increased risk of choriocarcinoma in the presence of active trophoblastic disease.

Reports on the COC include associations with a long list of 'minor' side-effects such as nausea, depression, weight gain, bloatedness, breast tenderness and lassitude that have not reached significance in good quality clinical trials. These complaints are often present in people taking the inactive preparation in trials that include a 'placebo' arm, that is, the comparison with an inactive treatment. This, of course, would not be ethical in trials of contraception, so it is impossible to compare these complaints with those arising in people receiving an inactive treatment.

Miscellaneous myths and why they are untrue

- *Women get more drunk if they are on the Pill.* There are contradictory papers on this — one suggesting that alcohol is cleared more slowly in users of COCs, another that women recover more quickly! It is wise advice not to drink too much — women may have sex unwisely or vomit after taking their Pill, both of which put them at risk.
- *Women should not take the Pill if they are flying.* Flying, especially if combined with sitting in a confined space (an airline seat), dehydration and the lower oxygen concentration in an aircraft, increases the risk of thrombosis. Give advice to reduce the risk by frequent activity, adequate non-alcoholic fluids, and do not risk pregnancy (which has a higher risk of thrombosis) by stopping the Pill.
- *The metal coil will set off the metal detector in airports.* Fortunately this does not happen.
- *'My friend said her coil came out when she and her boyfriend were trying out some new positions.'* There is no evidence that an IUD that is correctly positioned will be expelled during sexual athletics, only if it is already on its way out.
- *Sterilisation gives you heavy periods.* The period loss will be increased if the woman stops a hormonal method of contraception that had previously reduced her loss. So the periods revert to what they were like naturally.

Emergency contraception

General information   1

Emergency contraception comes in two forms in the UK:

- a pill method
- an intrauterine device.

Emergency contraception is popularly called the 'morning-after pill', but this term is misleading as the pills can be taken up to 72 hours after unprotected sex. The standard advice is for one pill to be taken immediately and another after 12 hours. Intrauterine devices can be used after this time, so refer to a provider if the time limit has been exceeded or if the woman prefers to use an IUD.

In the UK prescriptions or supplies of levonorgestrel (Levonelle-2) obtained from a GP or FP clinic are free. Pharmacists may charge (around £24 in the UK) for advice and supply without a prescription. In some areas pharmacists can advise and supply emergency contraception without charging the clients, depending on local arrangements.

Rarely, nausea or vomiting may occur. If vomiting occurs within three hours of taking the pills, the woman should take another pill. Always advise the use of condoms (or avoidance of sexual intercourse) until the next period. Give advice about the risk of STIs as protection against these has also been lost. Make sure that the woman knows that the method can fail and that she should seek advice if her next expected period does not arrive.

Advise that the woman should contact the FP clinic, practice nurse or GP if:

- the next period has not occurred by seven days after the expected date
- the period is unusually light, or shorter than usual
- there is any lower abdominal pain (in case of ectopic pregnancy).

Carry out a pregnancy test if there is *any* suspicion that the emergency pills have not worked as the failure rate is around 5% mid-cycle.

Most FP clinics and GP surgeries make special arrangements for seeing people for emergency contraception quickly. Providers need to ensure that these arrangements are clear to users and well advertised.

When is emergency contraception needed?

There is no day of the menstrual cycle when a woman can be *certain* that   2
unprotected sexual intercourse (UPSI) will not result in pregnancy, particularly if she has irregular periods or is unsure when her last period occurred.

Unprotected sexual intercourse includes any contact between semen (ejaculate) and the vagina when an effective method of contraception is not being used, or has not been used correctly. This includes damage to a condom, the condom coming off too early or incorrect use of a condom or other barrier method.

Missed pills are a frequent cause of anxiety. The reliability of contraceptive protection is reduced for COCs after:

- two or more pills are missed from the first seven pills in a packet
- four or more pills are missed after the first seven days of pills have been taken.

If two or more combined pills are missed from the last seven pills in a packet, emergency contraception is not necessary as long as the pill-free break is omitted, i.e. the woman starts her next packet of pills the day after finishing the current packet.

For progestogen-only pills, emergency contraception is needed if no extra precautions (such as a barrier method) are used when having sexual intercourse when one or more pills are taken more than three hours after the usual pill-taking time, or forgotten completely.

Emergency contraception may be needed if an IUD is completely or partially expelled or if the removal of an IUD is regarded as necessary within the seven days after sexual intercourse.

Failure rates of emergency contraception

Figures from the WHO studies in various countries (published in the *Lancet*) gave increasing pregnancy rates the longer the time after UPSI.[11] Rates of protection against pregnancy were:

24 hours or less after UPSI	95%
25–48 hours after UPSI	85%
49–72 hours after UPSI	58%.

Intrauterine devices are much more effective with a protection rate of 99.9%. An IUD can be inserted to prevent pregnancy up to five days after the expected time of ovulation. This is usually 14 days before the next period, so the time limit is usually 19 days after the first day of menstrual bleeding in a 28-day cycle. It can be used as a continuing method of contraception, if that is what the woman wants, or removed at the next menstrual period.

Multiple episodes of unprotected intercourse, even within the time limits, will increase the risk of pregnancy.

2

Timing of the next period after oral emergency contraception

Most women start their next period within three days of their expected date, **2** some start early, some are up to seven days or more late. It is important to advise women to return for a pregnancy test if they are more than seven days late with their expected next period. Bleeding between periods may sometimes occur before the next period after hormonal emergency contraception.

Some bleeding between menses is common after IUD insertion. There is no evidence that the timing of the next period is altered after post-coital insertion.

Other considerations

Larger doses of hormone are necessary to obtain the same blood levels for **3** patients who are taking any medication that raises hepatic enzyme levels (e.g. phenytoin or carbamezepine for epilepsy). Most providers give either three pills (two pills followed by one pill 12 hours later) or four pills (two pills followed by two pills 12 hours later). The best regime is not known. Consider an IUD if rifampicin is being taken because it is such a potent long-lasting enzyme-inducer.

Another method of contraception such as a barrier method (condom or cap) or abstinence should usually be advised until the onset of the next period. Opinions vary as to how to restart the COC or POP pills after the use of emergency contraception. There is no evidence to guide us. Most practitioners advise patients to continue with the pack with additional precautions for seven days as for the missed pill rules (see later in this section), but some feel happier advising the use of other methods until the next period arrives and then restarting with a new pack.

Most people take an individual decision based on the relative risks of each method and the number of remaining pills in the pack. However, there is no evidence that taking the COC or POP when pregnant increases the risk of fetal malformations if the woman decides to continue with an initially un-desired pregnancy.

The WHO has published the results of a large trial comparing the efficacy of 10 mg mifepristone, 1.5 mg levonorgestrel and two doses of 0.75 mg levon-orgestrel 12 hours apart used up to 120 hours after a single act of unprotected sexual intercourse. They reported no significant differences in efficacy between these three regimes. These findings suggest that the levonorgestrel dose does not need to be split and a single double dose would simplify treatment. However, these results must be interpreted with caution before any new general recommendation can be made.[12] The findings do make it simpler to advise a woman who would be outside the 72-hour limit with her second dose (give both together) or if she thinks she would forget the second dose. The WHO trial also showed that there was protection against pregnancy up to five days after exposure, although success rates fell the longer the interval was between exposure and taking the emergency contraception.

Risks of STIs

Pregnancy is only one of the risk factors as a result of unprotected intercourse. It also involves exposure to possible infection, so informed consent for screening is required, especially if an IUD is to be fitted. STIs will rarely be symptomatic by the time someone is seen for emergency contraception, if they become symptomatic at all (see Chapter 7).

If screening for infection is agreed, arrangements for contacting the woman with the results must be made. Many young people will not want postal contact at home, but can give the address of a trusted friend or a mobile phone number. If the woman will only agree that she makes contact herself for the results, you may be left with a considerable dilemma if she does not make contact and the results show that she has an infection.

People often feel that they cannot have an infection, that they would not have sex with anyone who they perceived as 'dirty' and that you are causing offence by suggesting it. Careful explanation of the invisibility of most infections, that anyone can carry an infection without knowing it etc. and allowing time to decide (or change from previously refusing) can all help to preserve self-esteem.

Accessing emergency contraception

It is embarrassing enough for anyone to attend a pharmacy or reception desk and blurt out that they need emergency contraception. It is particularly awkward if you belong to a cultural or religious group that would disapprove of sexual activity under the sort of circumstances that are likely to precipitate a need for emergency contraception. For example, if a couple are of different religions, but expected to marry someone of the same religious faith, a friendship that unexpectedly results in sexual activity may be even more of a disaster than usual. If the woman is from a culture in which premarital sexual activity is forbidden, she will be even more constrained to keep her need for emergency contraception well concealed. Other difficult scenarios include those where the woman does not wish to become pregnant, but the man would like her to be to prove his virility or position in his cultural group.

Opportunities to seek help from places where confidentiality is more likely to be achieved are needed. Concealment of the need for emergency contraception can be perceived as being more achievable in an anonymous clinic, distant general practice surgery or pharmacy in a town where the woman is not known. The main obstacle to all of these is the need to travel. Especially for young people in rural areas, the only transport may be with parents or friends of parents. Lack of knowledge of available sources of help in distant venues is also a deterrent. It is important for all those in contact with people at risk to have clear ideas of what help is available where, how and when it can be accessed and the standards of confidentiality offered.

Availability of counselling and supply of emergency contraception from pharmacies increase the access to the method and can reduce the delay before access. The pharmacists and their staff increase their knowledge of the local provision for contraceptive and sexual health advice and can pass on this information to their customers. If you know that a woman is seeking a supply from a pharmacy, it is sensible to check that she is aware of her risk of STIs and advise screening as necessary.

Pharmacists who have received training and are following a patient group direction (PGD – see p. 138) give advice in an area of the shop that is private. However there may be confidentiality problems while waiting because of lack of private waiting space, or when asking to see the pharmacist because of poorly trained or careless sales assistants. Attitudes of sales assistants sometimes also give rise to concern when judgemental attitudes are shown and the woman is made to feel cheap or stupid.

These attitudes can also be conveyed unconsciously by anyone in contact with people in this predicament. People can be made to feel that they have behaved irresponsibly, whereas they should be commended for seeking help after a mistake or misfortune. Even staff in medical establishments, who should be aware of their own attitudes, may project disapproval and irritation.

Many nurses have undertaken extra training and are able to advise and issue emergency oral contraception under PGDs. As part of maintaining standards of care, ensure that records include:

- date of last menstrual period
- usual cycle length
- date and time of unprotected sexual intercourse (UPSI)
- day of cycle of UPSI
- any other UPSI since last menstrual period
- options discussed (oral/IUD)
- any interacting medication (in case a higher dose is needed)
- current liver disease or history of porphyria (the only contraindications).

Counselling should include advice about:

- repeating the dose or considering an IUD if the pill is vomited up within three hours
- how the pills are thought to work
- the failure rates
- any side-effects to expect
- when to expect the next period
- doing a pregnancy test if the next period is not on time
- future contraception needs.

When issuing guidelines:

- negotiate the time of first and second dose and write them down
- go through a leaflet on emergency contraceptives with the patient
- make follow-up arrangements or advise return one week after expected date of next period
- record what emergency contraception has been given or prescribed.

Nurses may be available in walk-in clinics or at short notice in GP surgeries. Make a list of the local arrangements so that you can give advice to anyone who needs to know what is available and when.

Involving the man

All too often, emergency contraception is seen as the responsibility of the woman – she will be the one who gets pregnant! It is encouraging to see more males asking about the availability of emergency contraception, and this is the ideal time to talk about contraception and their responsibility for checking that it is in use beforehand. Discussion about how to negotiate the use of condoms (so important in a new relationship), and finding out what other contraceptive methods are in use, helps them to feel more confident and play an active part in taking responsibility. **2**

Practical and ethical issues

After ovulation, implantation occurs in the uterus after five days. Ovulation most frequently occurs about 14 days before the next menstrual period, so an **3**

IUD can be fitted to prevent implantation up to day 19 in a 28-day cycle. If the cycle is normally longer or shorter than 28 days from the first day of menstruation, then calculate the day of implantation as 14 days before the next expected period.

Theoretically, it should be possible to give oral emergency contraception up to five days after the expected date of ovulation. However, failure rates increase markedly if it is taken after the second day. Trials of administration up to five days have shown some effectiveness, but the numbers are small so an IUD is preferable (and more effective).

Some religious and cultural groups believe that life begins at fertilisation, and that methods of contraception that act after there has been a possibility of fertilisation are not permissible. During counselling the mode of action should be discussed – that the emergency contraception is to prevent implantation. If this is unacceptable to the beliefs of the woman, she will have to hope that she is not pregnant and wait until the next menstrual period to start on a more reliable method that works prior to fertilisation.

Contraceptive counselling

Getting to see a health professional[3]

This can often be the first hurdle, particularly for young people. The layout of a reception area may cause difficulties if patients at the desk can be overheard by others standing behind them. Clerks or receptionists often ask patients why they need an appointment so that they can be helpful in directing them to the appropriate person or clinic, or can make them an appointment of a suitable length. This can be very off putting if you are not very articulate, not sure how to ask for contraception or worried that someone might hear the reason for your attendance. Sometimes the receptionists have been placed in a difficult position because of decisions made by other members of the team who have not thought through the consequences of the receptionist having to ask intrusive questions. Structure your reception area to minimise embarrassment.

Small changes at the interface between the public and reception staff can make life more comfortable for both. The physical layout of the desk so that only one person is in front of the receptionist, with the others waiting some distance behind, is helpful. Using a roped-off queue (as used in many shops or railway stations) can prevent conversations at the desk from being overheard by the rest of the queue. A separate room for taking personal details is ideal. Some clinics ask the patients to complete their own personal details when they first attend. This could easily be modified so that patients complete the details on a computer screen (with access security procedures in place). However, those with literacy or language problems may have difficulties and need sensitive help.

Reception staff are the shop window of any clinic or practice. They need training and practice to feel confident at spotting the nervous patient who is unsure as to what or whom they wish to see. Use role-play or case scenarios to help with understanding why the difficulties arise and to rehearse ways of overcoming them.

Consider how to manage the needs of young people. They often need to be **2** seen urgently – to be protected that day. Frequently they have had difficulty accessing services at the clinic or surgery and will not want to be away from wherever they are supposed to be for long. However irritating it is for health staff (who bemoan the lack of planning by young people), it is a fact of life that *most* people do not plan sexual activity well in advance! Clinics at lunchtimes, immediately after school, Saturday clinics near shopping areas or clinics linked with other services all help to increase availability of contraceptives.

Older women may have special needs as well. They often want longer-acting methods of contraception and may have considerable problems in finding out where to obtain them and in attending. Often the longer-acting methods are only available from a surgery or clinic not in their immediate area, or held at a time, or on a day, that makes it impossible to attend because of work or family commitments. Part of the planning for contraceptive services in any area should take into account the need of the population for easily accessible venues (see Chapter 3).

Confidentiality must be assured at all stages of the process of obtaining contraceptive advice – fear of lack of confidentiality is one of the main reasons why young people do not attend for advice. Notices in a general practice or a clinic leaflet and posters help to spell out the importance of confidentiality. However, many people do not or cannot read notices, so that verbal reinforcement about confidentiality is essential. For example, staff need to tell patients who arrive with an accompanying person (as young people often do) that they can be seen on their own if they wish and that consultations are confidential to them. Many general practices inform young people and their parents that they can be seen on their own, and help young people to learn how to use the surgery by inviting them with a birthday card to a clinic for health advice.

Advice about how to obtain results of tests should always include the information that results will only be given to the person concerned and not to relatives or friends.

Patient group directions can be a good way of making sure that the needs of individuals can be dealt with promptly by whoever is available. If nurses are suitably trained and have a suitable PGD, they can assess risk factors and arrange for individuals to receive contraceptive care without the need for a return visit at another time. Not obtaining supplies of contraception at the first contact may mean that it is not used in the meantime – and then it may be too late.

Patient group directions should be drawn up in accordance with the national guidance for England,[13] Wales[14] and Scotland.[15] Included in the PGD are:

3

- the name of the organisation to which it applies
- the date it comes into effect and the date it expires
- a description of the contraceptive to which the PGD applies
- the type of health professional who may use the PGD (e.g. their qualifications or training required)
- the signature of the senior doctor or pharmacist and the representative of the health organisation involved
- a description of the circumstances in which the contraceptive can be used and those patients in whom it should not be used
- a description of the circumstances and arrangements for referral when appropriate
- details of how the contraceptive should be used and in what quantity and form it can be issued
- any warnings and side-effects
- what follow-up arrangements are to be made
- the nature of the record for audit purposes.

At least the nurse or pharmacist who will use the PGD, and the senior doctor giving authorisation for the PGD to be used, should sign the PGD. The nurse or pharmacist and the doctor need to be satisfied that the nurse or pharmacist is competent to carry out the PGD. In many areas there are guidelines about PGDs, such as requiring signatures from the primary care trust clinical governance officer and pharmacist in addition to the person authorised.

Discussing contraception

Sexual activity is enjoyable for most people, but contraception is hardly a feast of delight. Unless the advantages of avoiding pregnancy are obvious and people wish to use a particular method, it will be abandoned. So:

1

- Discover the individual's ideas about contraception and those of their partner.
- Use your check-list to select out the patient for whom that method would not be safe – a selected list appears p. 124.

- Negotiate an acceptable method.
- Teach the method using visual aids like leaflets and models.
- Arrange how to obtain supplies, advise when to return routinely and set up the safety net if things do not go to plan.

You can use any spare time for health promotion – advice on safe sex, smoking, diet and exercise etc. – but remember the prime concern is the provision of contraception.

You may want to think about who does what and how.[16] If contraceptive advice is done poorly and people leave with an inadequate grasp of how they are to use the method, or with unanswered (or not asked) questions about it, an unwanted pregnancy may result. If someone seeks information about contraception, the person being consulted must be properly trained so that accurate and up-to-date information and advice is given.

School-based sex education can be effective in reducing teenage pregnancy, especially when linked to contraceptive services. So consider how you can link with local schools and school nurses.

Contraceptives are highly cost-effective and can result in significant savings when used properly. Make sure that you have recent and accurate information yourself and that you have the skills and resources to help people learn how to use contraception effectively.

Increasing the availability of contraceptive clinic services for young people is associated with reduced pregnancy rates. Know about and publicise the availability of special teenage clinics. Encourage the development of youth-orientated clinics in places accessible to teenagers and open at times they can attend.

Contraceptive services should be based on an assessment of local needs (see Chapter 3) and ensure accessibility and confidentiality. People who live in rural communities or are disadvantaged by disability find it particularly difficult to access confidential contraceptive services.

When discussing contraception with young people:

- Discuss the guidelines on confidentiality with all young people.
- Always give the option of being seen alone.
- Follow up more frequently initially to build trust and confidence.
- Pelvic examination should only be considered if pathology is expected.
- Know the local procedure for child protection in case you learn that a young person is at risk of suffering or significant harm.
- Know and follow the 'Fraser guidelines' for advice and prescription for the under-16 year olds (see p. 108).

Look back at the section on 'Access and availability arrangements' (p. 105) to think about how cultural and religious differences affect the way in which contraception is chosen or used.

Specific advice on individual methods

After discussing the points for and against the chosen method, check that there are no contraindications to use (see p. 124). Then make sure that the individual understands how to use the method.

Combined oral contraceptives

Most people are generally uninterested in the long-term effects of COCs, but you should always ask if they have any worries and discuss them seriously to prevent early discontinuation of their contraceptive.

If the woman can start on the first day of her period, she will have taken enough hormones to prevent ovulation in the first pack. If she starts later she will need to take the COC for at least seven days before she is safe. After a first-trimester miscarriage or termination (first 12 weeks) she should start without delay, but in the mid-trimester and after delivery (if not breast-feeding) delay until the 21st day after delivery. This avoids the increased post-delivery thrombosis risk, but starts the hormones in sufficient time to prevent the first ovulation. If she is breast-feeding then a progestogen-only method is preferable.

Build in the safety net of what the woman should do if she experiences any major change in general health or has any problems that she is unsure about.

Missed pill advice needs frequent repetition. Use a leaflet like the example given in Figure 6.1 to reinforce your advice.

Discuss with a young woman who is living with her parents where she will keep her pills. If she has to conceal them from other family members she may be more likely to forget them. Building in reminder mechanisms such as keeping the packet with her clean underwear, or her toothbrush, may aid regular pill taking.

Ensure that she knows she should seek urgent advice if she has:

- sudden severe chest pain, breathlessness or cough with bloodstained sputum
- severe pain in the calf of a leg that persists or is accompanied by swelling
- severe stomach pains

- unusual severe or prolonged headache, visual loss, marked numbness or weakness affecting part of the body, disturbance of hearing, speech, balance, or a seizure
- hepatitis or jaundice.

Any of these may mean that oestrogen must be stopped and not used in the future. This is a major disadvantage for a young woman, so ensure that a clear diagnosis of the episode is made. Many people have been denied an excellent

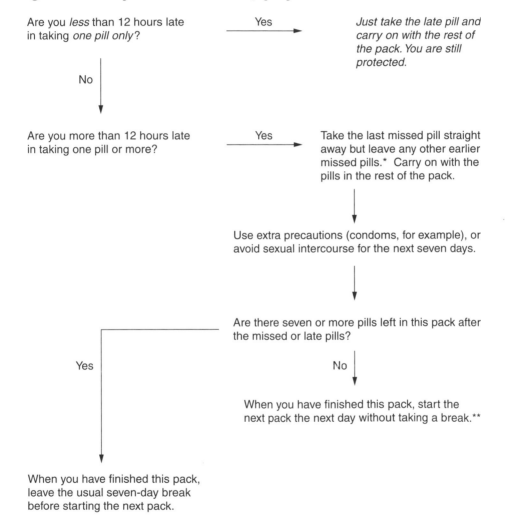

Figure 6.1   Advice on missed pills in a 21-day pack of contraceptive pills.

method of contraception because they have been advised to stop the COC for what sounds in retrospect like cramp in the calf.

Emphasise the dangers of lengthening the pill-free week. By the end of the pill-free week follicles may only be a couple of days away from being ripe enough to release the ovum and only become quiescent on restarting the COC. Fortunately this degree of activity only occurs in a few women, but nearly a quarter of women show some ovarian follicular activity by the seventh pill-free day. Seven pills after this are required to return the ovary to full quiescence[17] – the basis for the advice to use added contraception or abstinence for seven days after a missed pill.

Discuss interactions with other medication. Antibiotics may reduce the absorption of oestrogen, so advise the woman to take extra precautions while on antibiotics and for seven days afterwards. If on long-term antibiotics, the gut flora return to normal after about two weeks, so no extra precautions are needed after three weeks of use. Some anticonvulsants (phenytoin, carbamazepine, topiramate and barbiturates) and St John's Wort increase liver enzymes and reduce the effectiveness of hormonal medication. In that case, shorten the pill-free interval to five days, or give three packs continuously without a break (tricycling) or increase the dose of oestrogen to 50–90 micrograms. Use alternative methods if more potent liver enzyme-inducers such as rifampacin or rifabutin are being given. Check with a specialist if other less familiar drugs are being given, especially for new HIV treatments.

Some pills are produced in an everyday package with dummy pills for the seven pill-free days. These have not been very popular in the UK, mainly because of the risks associated with missed pills around that hormone-free week and the complicated instructions needed if pills are forgotten or vomited. Triphasic (with three sets of pills of differing strength) or biphasic (with two sets of pills of differing strength) pills need more careful explanation with a demonstration pack. The woman may be put at risk of breakthrough ovulation if she takes one pack immediately after another because of the drop in hormone level. Postponing a withdrawal bleed for a holiday, or if a pill has been missed in the last week, needs careful explanation about which pills to select to maintain the same level of hormones.

Progestogen-only pill

Advise women to take the POP every day at the same time. Help them to decide what is the best time for them. Blood levels will be highest about three hours after taking it and then gradually fall, so the worst time to take the POP is just before expected intercourse which, for many people, will be at night or

2

the early morning. Taking the POP at lunchtime or teatime is a good choice, but any time that can be regularly remembered is better than an imposed solution. Some women use alarm watches to remind them.

Forgotten pills should be taken as soon as possible afterwards, but extra precautions against pregnancy should be advised if the POP is forgotten for more than three hours. Standard advice (to harmonise with that for COCs) is for the woman to use extra precautions (i.e. abstinence or condoms) for seven days. Interactions with hepatic enzyme-inducing drugs are the same as for COCs, but antibiotics have no effect on absorption and the blood levels.

Irregular light bleeding is very common with progestogen-only contraception, especially the POP. Most people can cope with this provided they are reassured that it is normal.

POPs are particularly suitable for those few women with health risks. Although people with diabetes can take the COC, they may have an increased cardiovascular risk with oestrogen and they usually have a regular lifestyle well suited to taking the POP. People with mobility problems, such as those in wheelchairs, can safely avoid the increased thrombosis risk associated with oestrogen by taking the POP.

The POP is particularly suitable for women with good memories and regular lifestyles and for those with contraindications to oestrogen. See p. 124 for cautions about use.

The POP works by keeping the cervical mucus in the post-ovulatory state when sperm find it difficult to penetrate. The endometrium is thinner and scantier irregular periods usually occur. In some women ovulation will be inhibited and these women usually have amenorrhoea. Ovarian cysts can develop and cause pain, but usually resolve spontaneously. The risk of breast cancer is thought to be of the same order as for COCs and very small.

Be cautious about the use of progestogen-only methods in obese women (with a basal metabolic index of more than 30) who have an increased thrombosis risk with oestrogen. A woman who weighs over 70 kg appears to have a higher failure rate for some progestogen-only methods. Although this has not been demonstrated with the POP, some experts advise two pills daily (although unlicensed).

Bear in mind that many of the exclusions for the POP have been drawn from extrapolation of evidence about COCs and that you may need to seek expert advice in difficult clinical situations. The evidence is unsatisfactory[18] for any need for caution in patients with thromboembolism, hypertension, diabetes mellitus and migraine.

A newer POP containing desogestrel (called Cerazette in the UK) has been shown to inhibit ovulation in 97% of cycles. This should reduce the failure rate and increase the length of time before its efficacy diminishes after a forgotten pill. In some countries, it has obtained a licence giving the information that

3

additional precautions are only required if it has been forgotten for 12 hours (like the COC), but the licence in the UK is the same as for other POPs – additional precautions after it has been forgotten for three hours.

Injectable contraceptives

Give the injection within the first five days after the first day of the period and continue at 12-week (Depo Provera) or eight-week (Noristerat) intervals. **2**

Counselling about the usual infrequent or absent periods and the management of early irregular bleeding is important for good continuation rates. You must ensure that women have had ample opportunity to discuss any fears or queries about the method before giving an injection – the user cannot discontinue it if she has second thoughts later! Noristerat is only licensed in the UK for short-term use but is often used long term for those people who prefer it, perhaps because of the lesser risk of weight gain or the slightly different side-effect profile of norethisterone. Most women prefer the less frequent injections of Depo Provera.

Consider reducing the interval between injections if a woman often attends late for her injection. The World Health Organization advises that either the Depo Provera or Noristerat injection can be given up to two weeks late, but the licence for Depo Provera in the UK gives a leeway of only 12 weeks and five days. After that you might offer emergency contraception if the woman has had unprotected intercourse. Establish that pregnancy has not occurred before restarting the injection.

To manage bleeding problems with injectable contraception:

- clarify extent of bleeding
- consider other causes (chlamydia, cervical ectopy etc.)
- within four to eight weeks of last injection, consider COC for 21 days*
- if eight or more weeks since last injection, consider repeat injection*
- consider alternative methods of contraception if the bleeding is unacceptable.

Injectable contraceptives have no appreciable effect on the risk of thrombosis or a rise in blood pressure levels. It is suggested that they can be used in women with focal migraine[19] (who must avoid the COC). **3**

About 10% of women on Depo Provera stay the same weight and between 20 and 25% lose weight. It is common to gain some weight – the mean weight gain after 12 months is 2 kg, and 9 kg after 5.5 years, slightly more than the

---

*These regimes have no specific evidence to support them but are commonly used.

average over this period of time in this age group. Noristerat users seem to have comparatively less weight gain, but good evidence is lacking.

The concern that bone density might be reduced in long-term users of Depo Provera has been partially allayed by recent studies showing only small differences between users and the normal population mean. However, the COC would be protective for those at extra risk of osteoporosis if there are no contraindications to the use of oestrogen. Particularly in young women before the optimum bone mass is achieved at about 19 years of age, Depo Provera may be better used as a short-term method. Implants of progestogen do not seem to affect bone mass and may be a better choice for teenagers who are forgetful but need excellent contraception. If Depo Provera is the first choice of an individual, it may be preferable to start with that, but reconsider later if that person is at higher risk of low bone mass (a smoker, a diet low in vitamin D or calcium, little exposure to sunshine, low levels of exercise or medication affecting bone density).

The evidence concerning return to full fertility after Depo Provera is discontinued has recently been updated.[19] It used to be thought that return to full fertility was considerably delayed. However, recent studies show no delay once the effect of the last injection is eliminated (i.e. after 12 weeks). Comparative studies between the COC pill, the IUD and Depo Provera give a delay to first ovulation of less than 30 days for all of them. This has important implications for reinstated fertility if the woman is late attending for her next injection.

Progestogen implants

Implanon has only one rod (about the size of a hairgrip) so that insertion and removal are easier. It can be felt under the skin, but is less visible than the previously used implant Norplant (now discontinued) as it lies in the groove between the muscles. Good counselling about progestogenic side-effects, especially the irregular bleeding, reduces removal rates. Blood levels are similar to the progestogen-only pill, and side-effects are about the same, but without the need for a good memory!

Implanon is inserted just under the skin on the upper arm under local anaesthetic with a special introducer. Training for insertion and removal is available from centres that fit Implanon or by contacting the manufacturer. It should be inserted within five days of the first day of the period or while other reliable contraception is being used. It can remain in place for three years and then be removed under local anaesthetic by making a small cut in the skin and pulling out the plastic carrier rod. Another implant can be inserted in the other arm on the same occasion to continue the contraceptive effect.

Intrauterine devices

Copper-bearing IUDs appear to act mainly by blocking fertilisation. Sperm **3** transport is impaired and studies show that viable sperm are hardly ever found in the upper genital tract compared with other methods in sexually active women. The secondary protection from implantation blocking rarely has to come into action except when used for post-coital protection.

Pre-insertion counselling should cover the advantages as well as how to recognise the signs of expulsion, perforation, infection and ectopic pregnancy. Modern devices cause only a small increase in the length and heaviness of the regular menstrual loss, but irregular spotting is quite common in the first few months.

The risk of chlamydial infection and of pelvic infection is increased in the young and in those with more than two partners in the last 12 months. Consider taking swabs (with informed consent) before fitting an IUD, especially in higher-risk patients (see Chapter 7 on sexually transmitted infections). The risks of infection with an IUD occur mainly in the first three weeks. Bacteria from the vagina may be taken into the uterus and cause endometritis or salpingitis during the fitting of the device. A sexual history and an estimate of the risks of changes of partner must be balanced against the effectiveness and ease of the method.

The choice of IUDs[20] in general practices may be limited by which ones are on the drug tariff. Devices that have less than 300 mm surface area of copper have a higher pregnancy rate than those with more copper. The Copper T380 series has low pregnancy rates, with the Multiload 375 a close second. T-safe Cu380A is now available in clinics and for use in general practices. The Nova-T380 is identical to the previous Nova-T200 except for extra copper on its stem, but should give lower pregnancy rates because it has more copper. The confusing names for these devices mean that you should inspect the pack carefully before fitting and record the type of device carefully. Make sure that you are aware of the different methods of insertion for each type of device.

The Flexi-T300 is introduced into the uterus with a simple push–pull action like the Multiload. Gynefix is a frameless device of copper tubes fixed into the fundus of the uterus with a knot and requires special training to fit. New IUDs are being developed with similar technology.

All of these devices are usually removed and refitted after five years (except the T-safe Cu380A which has a licence for eight years). However, if the woman had the IUD fitted after the age of 40 years it is normally removed after the menopause is definite (conventionally regarded as one year without periods after 50 years, or two years without periods before the age of 50 years). Too frequent removal and refitting increases the risk of infection, expulsion and failure.

Nova-T200 or the Multiload 250 are usually regarded as suitable only for short-term use because of their slightly higher pregnancy rate, and will eventually be discontinued.

The intrauterine system (IUS) Mirena

The failure rate is given as 0.2 per 100 women years. The IUS is a T-shaped **3** device with progesterone loaded on the upright stem. The main effects are to reduce the endometrial thickness and maintain the cervical mucus in its post-ovulatory thickened state. Menstrual flow is markedly reduced, making it an ideal contraceptive for a woman who usually has heavy loss.

Counselling before insertion should include advice about the expected menstrual pattern – frequent, sometimes continuous, light bleeding in the first three to six months settling to very light occasional loss or amenorrhoea. Side-effects due to the progesterone, such as acne and bloating, can also occur in the first few months but usually settle down as the blood level falls to below a third of the POP. Functional ovarian cysts may occur but usually resolve spontaneously.

Only fit the IUS if you have been trained as it has a different type of insertion technique to other IUDs. The full efficacy of the IUS occurs once the progesterone has had its effect. There will be a delay after fitting before full efficacy is achieved so the IUS is not licensed for post-coital contraception, and you should insert it within the first seven days after the onset of the period.

Cost-effectiveness of IUDs and the IUS

It makes sense to stock a limited number of contraceptive devices, both from **3** the point of view of becoming expert at fitting certain devices and because savings can be made by obtaining a discount by purchasing larger numbers of one type. Balance this by stocking enough variety to suit most patients and the needs of the clinicians fitting the devices.

The T-safe Cu380A, Multiload 375 and Flexi-T are almost the same cost in the UK (between £8 and £9 each, 2003 prices), but the T-safe Cu380 can be left in place for eight years. The Nova-T380 is more expensive (around £13.50, 2003 prices). Gynefix is about three times the cost of a T-safe Cu380A and should perhaps be a second-line device for patients who have had problems with pain, bleeding or expulsion with previous types of IUD.

A Mirena IUS is even more expensive at around £90 (2003 prices), but if it is replacing sterilisation is probably cost-effective. It is commonly indicated as treatment for problems such as heavy bleeding when additional costs would otherwise be incurred.

Resuscitation requirements

Severe pain or vasovagal collapse is rare but usually associated with dilatation of the cervical canal. Occasionally IUD insertion may provoke epileptic fits. The assistant to the person inserting the device needs to monitor the general condition of the woman. A light finger on the pulse while distracting the patient's attention with small talk is very useful.

If a woman develops faintness or slowing of the pulse during insertion of the device:

1 stop and raise the end of the couch
2 give oxygen through a face mask
3 support the chin to maintain a clear airway
4 monitor the patient's breathing, pulse and blood pressure.

If the woman does not recover rapidly, remove the IUD and consider giving atropine 0.5 mg slowly, intravenously, if a very slow pulse rate (under 45/minute) persists.

If the woman becomes unconscious maintain her airway, breathing and circulation until she is transferred to hospital by ambulance.

You should keep your own resuscitation skills refreshed and not be attempting to insert IUDs without an assistant also trained in resuscitation. Oxygen, a mask and an airway should be in the room where IUDs are fitted. You should also have a standard resuscitation drug box containing:

- adrenaline 1 in 1000 solution (1 mg in 1 ml) for allergic reactions
- atropine 0.5 mg for bradycardia (pulse rate persistently less than 45/minute)
- diazepam 10 mg in rectal suppositories for persistent epileptic fits.

If you are confident in your ability to cope with an emergency, you will provide the correct, calm and unhurried atmosphere that does much to prevent emergencies happening! Build in refresher courses on resuscitation on a regular cycle for all staff so that this uncommon occurrence does not provoke a panic reaction.

Condoms

You should be aware of the types available. Different sizes and shapes suit different sizes and shapes of men. Know where they can be obtained free to the user (e.g. community clinics) and other sources of supply. It is useful to have some idea of how much they cost to the public as well. Recommend them additionally for protection against infection to those who are likely to change partners. Discuss with people how they can negotiate the use of condoms with a partner, and how to obtain emergency contraception in the event of a failure in use.

Health professionals and providers of condoms need to be comfortable dis- **2** cussing how a condom should be used, and in suggesting ways in which it can be incorporated into love play. Advice on using water-based lubricants (not lubricants containing oil as that can weaken the latex) can reduce tearing and irritation as well as increasing sensitivity.

A proportion of both men and women dislike any form of barrier – condoms or **3** diaphragms (see below). They feel that this distances them emotionally from their partner or that it reduces sensitivity so that pleasure is diminished. However, some of the expressed dissatisfaction with barrier methods is due to myth rather than personal experience. Many of those who refuse to use barrier methods have never tried them and use the lack of sensitivity as an excuse to cover up other concerns. They have fears of losing the erection, of appearing foolish (because of lack of skill in putting it on) or that the partner will think that they are afraid of catching an infection.

Others welcome a method that reduces the messiness of ejaculation, or even welcome the emotional sense of distance that barriers produce, and may have difficulties if they then cease to use the barrier with changes of method or a desire for pregnancy.

Some people will object to them on religious or cultural grounds. This can sometimes be a defence against discussing them in case the man reveals ignorance about condoms. Sensitive discussion can disentangle which is the real reason.

Diaphragms and caps

A diaphragm fits across the upper part of the vagina from the ledge above the **3** pelvic bone to the back wall of the vagina. A cervical cap covers just the cervix and comes in different shapes to fit various types of cervix from conical to almost flat.

Having to have a diaphragm or cap fitted involves a vaginal examination and this may deter some people. The diaphragm or cap must always be used together with a spermicide. Good teaching and practice are essential to ensure that the diaphragm and pool of spermicide cover the cervix. Health professionals who fit cervical caps should have practical training so they are competent to fit them accurately and are able to choose the right type for each individual.

Diaphragms and caps should be put in before sexual intercourse and left in for at least six hours afterwards to ensure that no live sperm can access the cervical canal after removal. Most women put in the diaphragm before going to bed and take it out either the following morning (if they had sexual intercourse at the beginning of the night) or at lunch-time or the following evening (if they had sexual intercourse in the morning). When not in use, the diaphragm or cap should be washed, dried and checked for damage before being stored in a protective case.

The degree of organisation and forward planning required for reliable use makes diaphragms or caps a more suitable choice for those in stable, long-term relationships. Patients also require access to (preferably private) washing facilities and convenient storage.

Sterilisation

In the UK almost 30% of all couples and almost 50% of those over 40 years of age use either male or female sterilisation as their method of contraception.[21] Vasectomy is very widely used throughout the world, especially in developing countries.

Female sterilisation

Female sterilisation is achieved by blocking both the fallopian tubes that transport the egg to the uterus. It requires an operation to visualise them inside the abdominal cavity. In the UK this is usually done using a flexible tube called a laparoscope, which is introduced through a small cut in the abdominal wall under a general or local anaesthetic. Clips or rings are put onto the tubes to close them up. Usually the woman does not need to stay in hospital overnight. She can return to her normal work as soon as she is comfortable, usually after a few days. If it is impossible to see the tubes clearly through a laparoscope, the woman may need to have a laparotomy – a longer cut in the abdominal wall. This is more likely if she has had operations or infections in that area before or if she is obese. It is important to make sure that the woman is not already in the early stages of pregnancy before the procedure is done and she should continue using a reliable method of contraception until the next period.

Ensure that the woman understands that sterilisation is a permanent procedure. Although it is technically possible to reverse it, success rates are variable and ectopic pregnancy more likely. She should know what to expect and also be aware of the possible risks of the procedure.

Sterilisation can be done at any time of the menstrual cycle. Do a pregnancy test before operating if there is any doubt about the degree of protection afforded by the method of contraception. Contraception, including the COC, should be continued until the menstrual period following the operation.[22] Most women return to work within two days. If a laparotomy has been done, heavy lifting should be avoided for three weeks and the woman will take longer to get back to work. Female sterilisation is effective from the time of the next menstrual period and sexual activity can be started as soon as the woman feels comfortable.

Do not take out an IUD at the time of operation if the woman has had inter- **3** course in the last seven days in case a fertilised egg is already in the tube or the uterus. Remove the IUD with the next normal period to make sure that it is not forgotten. Absorbable stitches or plasters (steri-strips) are usually used to close the abdominal wound and it is usually fully healed by seven to ten days. Slight bruising and discomfort is usual for a few days. Some of the gas used to distend the abdomen (to get a good view of the tubes) may remain and give discomfort from distension or shoulder-tip pain for one to two days.

Infection or more severe bruising around the abdominal wound is unusual. Occasionally the bowel or other abdominal organs can be damaged during the surgery. This is usually recognised at the time, but anyone with unexplained pain or a temperature should be referred back to the operator urgently.

There is a small risk of death, less than eight per 100 000.

Ectopic pregnancy is a late risk — a large follow-up study in the USA found a rate of 7.3 ectopic pregnancies per 1000 sterilisations. Other failure of contraceptive effectiveness can also occur (two to three per 1000).[23]

Several studies have shown that amount or frequency of menstrual loss is not increased by sterilisation but may appear to be so if the woman has discontinued hormonal contraception that reduced the menstrual loss. However, this group of women may be less tolerant of heavy periods and request treatment more often than women who have not been sterilised.

Poor counselling before female sterilisation is a frequent cause for complaint. It is sensible to use a leaflet such as the one published by the FPA.[24] If you use one specifically designed for local circumstances, make sure that it has been properly piloted and checked so that you are sure it is comprehensive and can be understood by the majority of patients. A leaflet is an aid to counselling, not a substitute. A check-list of points to be discussed before referral is useful and could usefully be recorded in the patient's medical record:

- when current contraception should be stopped
- that the operation is intended to be permanent
- reversal may have to be funded privately
- the failure rate
- the ectopic risk

- that vasectomy (with its even smaller failure rate and lesser risk to health) has been discussed
- to seek advice if a period is missed or if the woman feels pregnant at any time after the sterilisation
- that surgical risks are small unless she is obese or has had previous surgery or infection in the pelvic area
- that it may be necessary to proceed to a laparotomy if there are difficulties.

Litigation has followed when women have been sterilised without adequate consent. Sterilisation should not be done during other operations without specific consent. Sterilisation done at the same time as a Caesarean section has a higher failure rate and is more likely to be regretted. The rate of requests for reversal is also higher the younger the woman at the time of sterilisation as her circumstances are more likely to change.

Sterilisation should never be done to 'save a marriage', or to improve sexual satisfaction or desire. It does not work and is frequently regretted if the partnership should subsequently fail. In some cultures, a woman can be rejected as a partner or wife if she is incapable of child-bearing. A few women will believe that they are no longer 'proper women' if sterilised and can suffer quite severe psychological after-effects.

Vasectomy

This operation involves the division or blockage of the vas deferens – the **1** tubes that take the sperm from the testis on each side. It is usually done under local anaesthetic in a clinic or in a general practice, but can be done under a general anaesthetic, although this increases the risk to health.

Make sure that both of the couple know that a vasectomy is not effective immediately and that other methods of contraception should be continued until he gets the 'all clear'. The man should produce a specimen of semen (ejaculate) for examination usually at 12 weeks and at 16 weeks after the operation to check that no sperm are present. Sperm are stored in the seminal vesicles, small glands in the prostate. These are nearer to the urethra (the pipe to the end of the penis) than the cut made for the sterilisation, so that they have to be emptied by ejaculations after the operation.

A history of previous surgery or infection in the inguinal area or having had **2** previous genital surgery may make the operation technically difficult. This may bias the operator towards doing the operation under a general anaesthetic. Otherwise the man should make an informed choice, bearing in mind the extra risks of a general anaesthetic. The referring doctor should examine the man' s genitals to rule out other abnormalities such as a hernia, varicocoele, cysts etc. that may need operative treatment in their own right.

The man is usually asked to shave himself in the inguinal and scrotal areas before the operation.

Advise him to wear a good supporting pair of underpants or a scrotal sports support after the operation for two to three days as this makes it more comfortable. Most men are able to return to work the day after the operation, but if he does heavy manual work, advise that he delays returning to work for three to four days to avoid bleeding from the operation site (and for comfort).

Some bruising around the operation site is usual, but about 1–2% of men will have more and a collection of blood (haematoma) may need evacuating.

About 5% of men will have a wound infection and require antibiotics.

Around 2% of men will not achieve a specimen free from sperm at 16 weeks. Check that this is not due to failure of ejaculation by the patient. A re-operation may reveal a dual vas deferens or other problem.

Late failure (many years later) rarely occurs (reports give an incidence of between one in 1000 and one in 2000).[21]

The man can resume penetrative sexual intercourse (with suitable contraceptive precautions) as soon as he is comfortable.

Small lumps may form at the site of the cut ends of the vas (sperm granulomas). These can be quite tender and may need removing. They also increase the risk of recanalisation. Cysts may form in the epididymis also. A few men develop chronic pain and tenderness in the scrotum that is made worse by sexual excitement and ejaculation. If chronic pain becomes a severe problem, some surgeons will cut out the epididymis and obstructed vas deferens but this does not always cure the pain.

After vasectomy, most men develop antibodies to sperm. This may cause problems with fertility later even if reversal is sought and is technically successful.

Research studies have not confirmed early concerns about links between vasectomy and cardiovascular disease, autoimmune diseases, endocrine disease or cancer.

Late failure of vasectomy requires sensitive handling. It often leads to accusations of infidelity and requests for paternity testing. If the paternity is accepted without question, some doctors will offer a re-operation without any examination of the semen in case this upsets the relationship. However, this course of action may store up trouble for later and you need to consider carefully with the couple (separately and together) what they wish to do.

3

Chronic pain after vasectomy is a problem in a small minority of men.[25] A study found that the prevalence of chronic testicular pain was 6% in men who had had a vasectomy compared with 2% who had not had a vasectomy. Occasional pain was even more likely in men who had had a vasectomy. It may not be cured by surgery and a few may have psychosexual problems. For most men it is not a significant problem, but it is worth warning men of its possibility.

Several large studies have refuted any link between vasectomy and diseases. A useful review of the evidence appeared in the *British Journal of*

98

General Practice.[26] Investigations have failed to confirm the hypothesis that auto-immune complexes produced after vasectomy might predispose men to a variety of diseases such as cardiovascular disease, diabetes, joint disease or multiple sclerosis. Large follow-up studies have not confirmed any increase in the number of men with testicular cancer after vasectomy. A number of research studies from the USA have suggested a link between vasectomy and prostate cancer, but a large follow-up study in India (where vasectomy has been very popular) refuted this. It was suggested that the USA studies were biased because of the interests of the urologists carrying out the vasectomies as they continued to follow up their patients with repeated prostatic-specific antigen tests, and may well have diagnosed prostate cancer in larger numbers of men than would otherwise be known (see the section on screening for prostate cancer in Chapter 5). The World Health Organization reviewed the evidence in 1991 and concluded that there was *no* biological plausibility for a link. The National Institute of Health in the USA endorsed the WHO findings in 1993. A review of the literature in 1998 concluded that there is unlikely to be any link between prostate cancer and vasectomy.[27]

Which method is best?

The best method of contraception is one that is used consistently whenever **1** sexual intercourse takes place. Most people will be healthy with no medical contraindications to any method. Help them to choose the method that they feel most comfortable about. Others with medical contraindications will have a more limited choice. Present them with the choices that they have and help them to select the best for them depending on their precise circumstances.

Further reading

Becoming more expert is often best done by experiential learning and by **3** discussing difficult problems with others. Background knowledge from books and journals can help in this process and form part of your reflection about your work. Some books that are particularly relevant to this section follow:

Chambers R, Wakley G and Chambers S (2001) *Tackling Teenage Pregnancy: sex, culture and needs.* Radcliffe Medical Press, Oxford.
Donovan C, Hadley A, Jones M *et al.* (2000) *Confidentiality and Young People Toolkit.* Royal College of General Practitioners and Brook, London.

Hughes L (2000) Developing primary care services for young people. *British Journal of Family Planning* **26**: 155–60.

Guillebaud J (1999) *Contraception: your questions answered* (3e). Churchill Livingstone, London.

World Health Organization (2000) *Improving Access to Quality Care in Family Planning*. WHO, Geneva.

See the Appendix for other sources of help, advice and reference.

References

1 NHS Centre for Reviews and Dissemination (1997) Preventing and reducing the adverse effects of unintended teenage pregnancies. *Effective Health Care Bulletin* **3** (1): 1–12.

2 Joint Guidance Group (1993) *Guidance Issued Jointly on Confidentiality and People Under 16.* BMA, GMC, HEA, Brook Advisory Centres, FPA and RCGP leaflet.

3 Donovan C, Hadley A, Jones M *et al.* (2000) *Confidentiality and Young People Toolkit.* Royal College of General Practitioners and Brook, London.

4 Barna D, McKeown C and Woodhead P (2002) *Get Real: sharing good practice in the provision of sexual health services for young people.* Save the Children, London.

5 Schott J and Henley A (1996) *Culture, Religion and Childbearing in a Multiracial Society.* Butterworth-Heinemann, Oxford.

6 Chambers R, Wakley G and Chambers S (2001) *Tackling Teenage Pregnancy: sex, culture and needs.* Radcliffe Medical Press, Oxford.

7 Unlinked Anonymous Surveys Steering Group (2002) *Prevalence of HIV and Hepatitis Infections in the United Kingdom.* Department of Health, London.

8 Belfield T (1999) *Contraceptive Handbook* (3e). Family Planning Association, London.

9 Guillebaud J (1999) *Contraception: your questions answered* (3e). Churchill Livingstone, London.

10 World Health Organization (2000) *Improving Access to Quality Care in Family Planning*. WHO, Geneva.

11 Task Force on Post-Ovulatory Methods of Fertility Regulation (1998) Randomized controlled trial of levonorgestrel versus the Yuzpe regimen of combined oral contraceptives for emergency contraception. *Lancet* **352**: 428–33.

12 von Hertzen H, Piaggio G, Ding J *et al.* (2002) Low-dose mifepristone and two regimens of levonorgestrel for emergency contraception: a WHO multicentre randomised trial. *Lancet* **360** (9348): 1803–10.

13 NHS Executive (2000) *Patient Group Directions (England) HSC 2000/026.* NHSE, Leeds.

14 National Welsh Assembly (2000) *Review of Prescribing, Supply and Administration of Medicines by Health Professionals Under Patient Group Directions (PGD).* National Welsh Assembly, Cardiff.

15 Scottish Executive Health Department NHS (2001) *Patient Group Directions.* http://www.show.scot.nhs.uk/sehd/mels/hdl2001_07.htm

16 Montford H and Skrine R (1993) *Contraceptive Care: meeting individual needs.* Chapman and Hall, London.

17 Korver T, Goorissen E and Guillebaud J (1995) The combined oral contraceptive pill: what advice should we give when pills are missed? *British Journal of Obstetrics and Gynaecology* **102**: 601–7.

18 Joint Formulary Committee (2002) *British National Formulary.* British Medical Association and Royal Pharmaceutical Society of Great Britain, London.

19 Bigrigg A, Evans M, Gbolade B *et al.* (1999) Depo Provera. Position paper on clinical use, effectiveness and side-effects. *British Journal of Family Planning.* **25**: 69–76.

20 Dennis J and Hampton N (2002) IUDs: which device? *Journal of Family Planning and Reproductive Health Care* **28** (2): 61–8.

21 Glasier A and Gebbie A (2000) *Family Planning and Reproductive Care.* Churchill Livingstone, London.

22 Royal College of Obstetricians and Gynaecologists (1999) *Male and Female Sterilisation: evidence-based clinical guidelines summary no. 4.* RCOG Press, London.

23 Kovacs GT and Krins AJ (2002) Female sterilisations with Filshie clips: what is the risk failure? A retrospective survey of 30 000 applications. *Journal of Family Planning and Reproductive Health Care.* **28** (1): 34–5.

24 Contraceptive Education Service (2002) *Sterilisation.* Family Planning Association, 2–12 Pentonville Road, London.

25 Morris C, Mishra K and Kirkman RJE (2002) A study to assess the prevalence of chronic testicular pain in post-vasectomised men compared to non-vasectomised men. *Journal of Family Planning and Reproductive Health Care* **28** (3): 142–4.

26 Macdonald SW (1977) Is vasectomy harmful to health? *British Journal of General Practice* **47**: 381–6.

27 Peterson HB and Howards SS (1998) Vasectomy and prostate cancer: the evidence to date. *Fertility and Sterility* **70**: 201–3.

7

Sexually transmitted infections

Background of sexually transmitted infections (STIs)

Common STIs in the UK

- Chlamydia: the commonest bacterial STI.   **1**
- Genital warts: Genital warts (HPV) are the commonest viral STI and also the commonest STI overall.
- Non-specific urethritis, gonorrhoea, genital herpes (herpes simplex virus) and trichomoniasis are all common.
- Syphilis is quite rare in the UK, but occasional outbreaks occur.
- HIV rates are going up.
- Crab lice (crabs) are not common but an indication that other STIs may be present.
- Hepatitis B rates are slightly decreasing but hepatitis C rates are still increasing.
- Some other infections may be seen rarely and some infections that occur at other body sites can be spread sexually sometimes.
- Other causes of genital soreness or discharge such as thrush (candida) and bacterial vaginosis are not classified as STIs.

Statistics about STIs

- Cases of *Chlamydia trachomatis* identified have doubled in the last six years.   **2**
  In 2000, genital chlamydial infection was the commonest bacterial STI seen, with 64 000 diagnoses made in England, Wales and Northern Ireland.
- Genital warts: there were 72 233 new episodes recorded in 1999 up from 70 460 in the previous year.
- Gonorrhoea cases recorded increased from 13 190 in 1998 to 16 470 in 1999.

- Genital herpes first-attack rates rose slightly from 17 098 in 1998 to 17 456 in 1999.
- Syphilis numbers rose from 138 to 217 between 1998 and 1999.
- HIV numbers increased from 2761 to 2942 between 1998 and 1999.
- Hepatitis B slightly decreased from 861 to 749 between 1998 and 1999 but hepatitis C increased from 4521 to 5768, perhaps representing the effect of immunisation against hepatitis B.

Some other infections that occur elsewhere in the body such as streptococcus (that usually causes skin and throat infections), or gut bacteria like *Escherichia coli* (*E coli*), can be spread by sexual activity. Molluscum contagiosum is a very common infection, especially in children, but can also be spread through sexual activity. Some other more unusual STIs may be seen occasionally in people returning from other countries.

Thrush is also known as candida, or candidiasis, and is not usually passed on from a woman to a man by sexual intercourse. It is a very common cause of vaginal discharge, soreness and itching.

Bacterial vaginosis is possibly even more frequently found in women with complaints of vaginal discharge.

Statistics on the incidence and prevalence of STIs are collected from GUM **3** clinics. Other people diagnosed in primary care (general practices or FP clinics) or in secondary care (hospitals) will not be included in these statistics unless they also attend a GUM clinic.

The statistics are already out of date by the time they are published. Look at http://www.phls.co.uk for weekly returns from GUM clinics and for full statistics from previous years.

Different rates of infection in various groups

There are differences in rates of infection: **2**

- in various ethnic groups
- between males and females
- between heterosexual and homosexual activity
- in younger and older age groups.

Beware of jumping to conclusions and stereotyping people by their age, appearance or culture. The types of people infected depend mainly on the number of partners they have and the type of sexual activity practised (the risk of infection increases the more partners they have) rather than on their ethnicity. If people have recently arrived from, or lived for any length of time in, a country where rates of infection are high, they are more likely to have been exposed to infection. For example, rates of HIV infection are high in Africa so someone who has had an immunisation, injection or sexual activity there may be more likely to have become infected.

Gender – being male or female – seems to affect rates of diagnosis rather than representing a true variation in prevalence. Females are more likely to be diagnosed with chlamydia without having any symptoms, or without symptoms that they recognise as being due to a STI, because tests are taken in the clinics and general practice surgeries that they attend for other reasons. Men are more likely to be diagnosed as a result of presenting with symptoms of penile discharge or painful urination – so STIs such as gonorrhoea are more likely to be diagnosed in men. Men can see warts on their genitals more easily than women can.

Rates are higher in urban areas and in young people, perhaps representing the greater number of sexual partners available and availability of transport.

Chlamydia

Regional variation may reflect the provision of diagnostic services as much as disease prevalence. Studies carried out in selected population groups indicate rates of anything between 2% and 12%. Higher rates were recorded in people attending GUM and termination of pregnancy clinics, and lower ones in primary care. The real rates in the population are likely to be higher than that recorded because the infection does not produce any symptoms in up to 80% of people – so they are not tested. Highest rates of diagnosis of chlamydia are seen in young people, particularly women in the 16–19 and 20–24 year age groups. In 2000, 1% of the 16–19 year female population of England, Wales and Northern Ireland was diagnosed with genital chlamydial infection at a GUM clinic. Higher rates within the 16–19 year olds are seen in some regions of the UK. In London, 1.4% of the 16–19 year old female population was diagnosed with genital chlamydial infection at a GUM clinic. Similar rates were also seen in other predominantly urban regions, such as Trent. (See Chapter 5 for information on screening for chlamydia in people who have no symptoms.)

Gonorrhoea

The rise in the number of cases of gonorrhoea has been largest in the youngest age groups – 16–19 and 20–24 years of age. The majority of cases identified have been in men, largely because women rarely have symptoms.

Syphilis

The rise in the numbers of new cases of syphilis that recently occurred was **2** mainly in men who have sex with men.

HIV

HIV infection is now identified more commonly in heterosexuals than in **2** homosexual men. Infection rates are increasing, perhaps due to a relaxation of the vigilance of people who believed that they were at risk and used condoms after publicity campaigns, but have now become complacent about the risk as it is no longer in the news.

The challenges of sexual health promotion

All STIs are commonest in the younger age groups. People beginning sexual **3** activity frequently change partners. It is difficult for people to believe that they have an infection when they have no symptoms or signs, so the potential for spreading STIs like chlamydia and gonorrhoea is considerable.

Studies have shown that there are a considerable number of people without symptoms, mainly under the age of 20, who are infected with genital chlamydial infection but would not generally be perceived as being at risk. Trials support the effectiveness of screening for chlamydial infection in people who have no symptoms. Tests have been developed that are highly sensitive (over 90%) and are suitable for use on urine samples. The urine samples need to be the first passed fraction of the urine, not mid-stream samples, to gather the organisms from the urethra.[1] The patient must not have passed urine for at least one hour before passing urine for testing or being swabbed. Most GUM clinics ask their patients not to pass urine for two hours before attending an appointment, but the optimum time is unknown.

More people are seeking diagnosis and treatment than previously, but provision of sexual health services is not keeping pace with the demand. The greater willingness of young people to discuss their sexuality needs to be met with an equally open reception by health professionals and others, so that the young people are not made to feel stigmatised. A more mobile population of people who are often separated from their families (and other social restraints) increases the risk of infection.

Use of condoms decreases the risk of an STI, but users of other methods of contraception often neglect to also use condoms, thinking only to protect themselves against pregnancy, not infection as well.[2]

Rates of STIs in homosexual males declined in the mid-1990s after targeted campaigns in the UK about safe sex, but rates have increased recently, showing that the message of safe sex has to be repeated. Part of the health promotion activity within the *National Strategy for Sexual Health and HIV*[3] includes media campaigns (see Chapter 1).

Risk of STIs

The risk of sexual activity is usually graded into:

- low or no risk:
  - masturbation
  - sex only with the same partner, who never has sex with anyone else
- medium risk:
  - using a condom for sex with other partners or with someone who has had other partners
- high risk:
  - having sex with someone who has had other partners without using a condom.

Negotiation of the level of sexual activity is always difficult. Anyone with a low opinion of themselves, or who thinks that sexual activity is the only way to 'keep' a partner, will not be able to express clearly what they want. Even when levels of self-esteem are high, someone saying that they want to use a condom, or want to avoid the exchange of body fluids, may be perceived by a partner as a rejection or a condemnation of their previous lifestyle. Help with assertiveness techniques and ways of broaching the subject need practice. In some cultures, it may not be possible for a woman to express her opinions or wishes.

- Low or no risk:
  - sexual activity with only the same partner ever, and that partner doing the same
  - sexual activity with no exchange of body fluids
  - masturbation.
- Medium risk:
  - always using a condom or effective barrier between someone and any partner.

- High risk:
  - sexual activity with more than one partner, or someone whose infection risk is unknown
  - exchange of body fluids with no barrier between someone and their partner.

There may be particular difficulties with negotiation about safe sexual practices when an imbalance of power is present, such as where there is a large age disparity. In some cultures and religions the wishes of the male partner take precedence and it can be impossible to request the use of a condom, even if one or both know that there is a risk from sexual activity with other partners.

3

- Low or no risk:
  - masturbation alone or with a partner (but making sure any cuts or grazes are covered by a waterproof plaster or wear latex gloves)
  - use of personal sex toys (but making sure that they are washed after each use in warm soapy water)
  - kissing on the lips with no exchange of saliva, or on the body
  - hugging, cuddling, body rubbing, sexual arousal fully clothed, licking food off each other, or other activities that do not involve exchange of body fluids
  - sensual body massage (but ensuring that oils do not come into contact with latex or rubber that they can weaken)
  - erotic fantasy either alone or shared
  - anything else that gives mutual pleasure by consent and that does not involve exchange of body fluids.
- Medium risk:
  - vaginal or oral sex with a condom
  - giving oral sex to a man but not taking the ejaculate into the mouth
  - oral sex with a woman during her period but using a protection between each other and the body fluids
  - oral sex with a woman not during her period
  - 'rimming' with the protection of a barrier, e.g. dental dam
  - 'wet' kissing (French kissing) with open mouths depends on the health of the lips and mouth – bleeding gums or ulcers, cut lips, cold sores etc. increase the risk
  - sharing sex toys after washing (remove the batteries first) and covering them with a fresh condom for each user
  - use of a sex toy in the vagina after using in the anus, with a fresh condom for each use.
- High risk:
  - vaginal or anal intercourse without a condom, including withdrawal (coitus interruptus)

- oral sex to a man and allowing the ejaculate into the mouth
- oral sex with a woman during her period (menstruation)
- unprotected 'rimming' (licking a partner's anal area)
- finger insertion with cuts or grazes or during menstruation
- getting human faeces or urine into the mouth
- sharing sex toys without a fresh condom
- unprotected sex with more than one partner after another, or without a change of condom.

Negotiating safe sex with a partner requires skill and may have to be learnt so that it can be approached without offending the partner. Imbalance of power between partners may make insisting on safer sexual practices impossible, or run the risk of physical, emotional or verbal abuse.

Health professionals need to discuss safer sexual practices with individuals and this can be tricky as well. When you ask people what they do, it is important to explain why you need to know and what risks they may be running. Giving examples often helps people to be more open about their sexual activities as they appreciate that you will not be shocked or judgemental. People will worry, too, that you will write down what they say and it will not be kept confidential — so discuss how that record will be kept confidential, and who needs to have access to that information.

The common myths about the spread of STIs and why they are wrong

- *Only 'that sort of person' gets a STI, not me.* Anyone can be infected.   **1**
- *You can always tell if someone is likely to have a STI.* Most people who have a STI look like everyone else.
- *You only get a STI if you sleep around.* It only takes one act of unprotected intercourse with someone who is infected to catch something.
- *You can only catch HIV if you are a homosexual.* More heterosexuals than homosexuals tested positive for a new infection with HIV in 2001.
- *You can get a STI from public toilets or using a bath after someone else has used it.* Most STIs are quite delicate outside the body and die quickly unless kept in a warm culture.

- *You will always know if you have caught something.* Many STIs do not produce   **2** any signs or symptoms, particularly in women.
- *You can't get an infection if you are using contraception.* Only a barrier method like a condom helps to prevent infection. The Pill does not give the same protection.

- *I always use a condom so I'm bound to be free from infection.* A condom helps but is not 100% safe.
- *Having sex with a teenager is much safer than with an older woman.* Rates of STIs are high in the 16–19 year old group.
- *HIV is the commonest STI.* In the UK it is not common. Chlamydia, genital warts and NSU are the most common, with gonorrhoea making a come-back bid recently.
- *Lesbians can't get STIs.* They can if they use any of the medium- or high-risk activities above.

- *If I'm told I have a STI and I've been with the same partner for six months, the partner must have cheated on me.* Many STIs can lie hidden inside the body cells, or in the vagina, without you knowing that they are there, e.g. many people have a wart virus without any visible warts. **3**
- *If I'm told I may have TV after a routine smear test, my partner must have been unfaithful.* Trichomoniasis vaginitis is sometimes identified wrongly on a cervical smear slide. It should always be confirmed with a proper test before treatment and contact notification.
- *Having a negative HIV test means that I'm all clear.* No test is 100% accurate and the result must be taken together with other evidence – like how long it is since exposure to the risk of HIV and what sort of risk it was.
- *Spitting can spread HIV.* No evidence has been recorded of anyone being infected in this way. Washing the spit off with soap and water if it hits you is all you need to do.
- *HIV can be spread by mosquito bites.* Mosquitoes do not inject you with blood, so cannot infect you with HIV.

Partner notification (contact tracing)

Why is partner notification needed?

The infection has been caught from 'someone else'. You want to make sure that 'someone else' does not give it back (causing reinfection), or give the infection to anyone else, and that he or she is also treated. Managing someone who has more than one *current* partner is likely to have the greatest impact on reducing the spread of infection. It may also help to identify the small networks of people who have the riskiest sexual lifestyles, so that education can target these groups. **1**

Referral to a GUM clinic and contact tracing is required if: **2**

- symptoms started after a recent change of partner, or intercourse with several partners, or an unknown partner

- recurrent or persistent symptoms occur despite simple investigations or treatments
- the partner also has symptoms
- symptoms or signs suggest involvement of other body systems, e.g. rash, joint pain, generalised enlarged lymph glands.

People with HIV are reluctant to disclose that they have the infection to others, suggesting that they expect harmful effects from disclosure. One study showed that 42% of people who had *not* told their partner(s) only used condoms some of the time – putting their partner(s) at risk. Another study showed that even after repeated individual counselling to encourage disclosure, 30% had not told previous partners and 29% had not told current partners after a six-month interval in which to do so.[4]

There is evidence that the detection and prompt treatment of chlamydial **3** infection, together with contact tracing of sexual partners, can reduce the subsequent risk of pelvic inflammatory disease, tubal infertility and ectopic pregnancy.[4] However, many women with chlamydia are often treated without any attempt to treat their partners, and they easily become reinfected. The same often happens when people are seen in clinics that are not set up to trace partners – gynaecology and urology particularly, but general practice and FP often have the same difficulty. It has been shown that many women who have tests taken before a termination of pregnancy (when they have obviously had unprotected sexual intercourse) leave hospital before the results of the test are known. If they are treated anyway just in case, they become reinfected by their untreated partner shortly afterwards.[5]

How is partner notification usually carried out?

Partner notification is the process whereby the sexual partners of a person who **1** has a confirmed diagnosis of a STI are informed about their exposure to that infection.

Most people with a STI are referred to the GUM clinic where the health advisor arranges partner notification.

Partner notification can be done by:

- the person with the infection
- the clinic or person making the diagnosis
- an agency on behalf of the clinic or doctor
- outreach workers in the community (usually connected to the clinic) who do not disclose the name of the contact.

Preferably, people should be referred to a GUM clinic or other facility where **2** trained health advisors can undertake the contact tracing and arrange for treatment. People with a STI can go to any GUM clinic in the country for testing and treatment.

You should obtain consent and offer a choice of how contacts should be notified, especially if you cannot persuade people to attend GUM clinics:

- patient referral – index patients themselves notify their sexual contacts to advise them to seek treatment
- provider referral – the healthcare professional (or someone on their behalf) informs the sexual contacts anonymously that they should seek treatment
- conditional referral – the healthcare professional notifies the contact directly if the patient has not managed to do so after a specified number of days.

Usually the sexual contacts who are notified are:

- all sexual partners in the last four weeks of people with symptoms
- all sexual partners in the last six months, or the most recent sexual partner if none for that time or more, of people with no symptoms.

Take into account the cultural and religious attitudes of the client. It can be complicated to obtain consent for contact tracing when an infection has been acquired from a liaison not sanctioned by the group or religion.

It is often difficult to persuade people to attend GUM clinics. A decision may **3** have to be made to treat only the person attending and to rely on that person to urge their partner(s) to seek testing and treatment – a scenario that is doubtful! In that situation it must be the decision of that person, after being given full information, to put themselves at risk of reinfection. Provider referral (i.e. by the clinic or health professional) is usually more reliable than patient notification. It may be easier to negotiate a compromise – that the health advisor carries out the partner notification if the patient finds, after a set time, that they have not been able to tell the partner(s).

No specific method of contact tracing or partner notification has been shown to be definitely any more effective than another, but telephone reminders and contact cards have been found to be helpful. It is not known whether giving people the choice of the type of partner notification helps to increase the identification of contacts. Nor has there been any work comparing different groups of people, such as people with combinations of STIs or from different settings. There is a suggestion from some research work that educational videos or leaflets might help to increase disclosure.[4]

Relying on telephone contact might be ineffective or counterproductive in some groups. Telephone ownership is often temporary – mobile phones are

often only in the possession of many young people for short periods of time
because of financial difficulties or theft. Others may answer a telephone call
when people are living in parental or shared accommodation and confidentiality
is then compromised.

Identification and treatment of STIs

Making diagnosis and treatment available

It is important that an adequate but sensitive sexual history is obtained,   **1**
including the number and the gender of partners. Do not make assumptions
but ask open questions, so that the person who suspects they may have a STI
can gradually reveal information at their own pace. Refer back to Chapter 4 for
further details on how to take a sexual history.

Anyone who has:

- an unusual discharge
- irritation or a rash in the pubic area
- pain when passing urine
- lumps on the genital area
- ulcers or sores on the genitals
- pain in the genital area
- pain on sexual intercourse
- contact with sexually transmitted infection

should have a check-up to make sure that they do not have any of the STIs.

Some vaginal discharge is usual and normal. The amount and type varies
throughout the cycle from being very scanty just after the menstrual period,
through the thin (like egg white) and large amount around mid-cycle, to the
stage of being thick and easy to roll up into a ball after ovulation. Many
complaints about vaginal discharge are due to lack of information about the
variations during the cycle, and lack of being aware that increases in amounts
can be due to irritation from chemicals such as soaps or perfumes or from
pressure from clothes or seating. Persistent complaints of discharge in the
absence of other symptoms, signs or evidence of infection should make you
think about a possible sexual problem or a phobia.

The individual should make an appointment at the local GUM or sexual
health clinic. Women can usually also have some tests at FP clinics or at their
GP surgery. However, there are very few places as yet outside a GUM clinic
that can offer full screening for all STIs. It is important to note that if an
individual has been at risk from one STI then they could have caught other

infections. Tests for *all* STIs are essential if unprotected sexual activity has occurred, in order to rule out any infection.

Sexual partners should be treated at the same time, avoiding any sexual activities until treatment is finished.

The telephone or contact address of the GUM clinic is usually available from a hospital switchboard, or from any NHS healthcare providers such as clinics and GP surgeries. In some areas the contact arrangements are on display in public toilets and in telephone directories, and many resource booklets for young people include the telephone number and address.

The new name for these clinics causes some confusion. They were previously known as 'special' or 'VD' (venereal disease) or sometimes 'STD' (sexually transmitted disease) clinics – and by a lot of nicknames such as the 'clap clinic', the 'back lane' clinic etc. Access to these clinics varies across the country and new users often find it difficult to know what is available. Healthcare workers and people working with teenagers should make sure that they know where they are, and how people can be seen. Some clinics have open access, others require appointments to be made by telephone. Some are open in the evening, others from 10 a.m. to 5 p.m. Some of the clinics now have a seamless one-stop service together with contraceptive clinics and are often known as 'sexual health clinics'. The GUM clinic may be on the same premises as contraceptive services to allow for easy transfers between the services.

What happens at a GUM clinic

The clinic will record a name and a date of birth, and will ask for a contact address so that results can be given (but clients do not have to give an address if they prefer not to). The medical records are kept separately from other hospital records and are confidential. By law, staff in a GUM clinic cannot tell a client what infection their partner has, or tell their doctor that they have attended, unless the client requests it. The clinic cannot give any information to other doctors, solicitors, insurance companies or the police without the consent of the client.

At the family planning clinic or GP surgery

After taking a sexual history, the health professional may ask the patient to go to the GUM clinic for full testing. The doctor or nurse may make arrangements to do the tests at the surgery or clinic. This is most likely if the history suggests that the complaints are likely to be due to thrush or bacterial vaginosis (which are not STIs) or if the diagnosis from taking swabs or urine samples is not complicated. Not all clinics and surgeries have the facilities for taking the full range of tests and the delays in transporting the samples may reduce the accuracy of the tests.

Identification of infection

If a discharge has increased in amount, has an unusual smell or a change in colour, the individual may have an infection. It is important to have this checked out as soon as possible so that it can be treated before it spreads. Common serious causes of an increased discharge in young people are trichomoniasis and gonorrhoea.

Over three-quarters of people with chlamydia do not know that they have any infection. Symptoms of burning on urination may be due to chlamydia, NSU, or to other non-STIs, although these are not common in young men.

Pain and small ulcers may indicate herpes simplex infection, but can also be due to other infections such as thrush.

Small lumps, either flat and shiny or looking like warts, can be due to wart viruses such as HPV.

People may feel reluctant to attend a GUM clinic, either because of perceived stigma ('I'm not that sort of person') or because of difficulties of attending. Many clinics do not have sufficient staff, premises or funding to open for more than restricted hours, often just during the daytime when many people are working or at school or college. Travel to GUM clinics, especially from rural areas, can be difficult for young people. They often cannot attend a clinic in a distant town without divulging to adult the reason for their need for transport. The disapproval that they encounter, or fear that they might find, is a potent deterrent to seeking advice.

At clinics and GP surgeries, staff may be less confident in taking an adequate sexual history or arranging suitable tests. In some areas, test equipment or laboratory testing is not available or limited in scope. The clinic or surgery may have difficulty in making arrangements to transport any samples, without delay, to a hospital laboratory. It is often better from the accuracy of the diagnosis point of view for patients to take themselves to the hospital to have samples taken, but access to a GUM clinic may be difficult (see above).

Common STIs

Trichomoniasis

The most frequent complaint in both men and women is of discharge, but between 15 and 50% of men have no symptoms and 10–50% of women are

2

also asymptomatic. Women also complain of itching, pain on passing urine or a smelly discharge. Although the discharge is classically described as frothy yellow or green, it is often variable both in consistency and colour.

In the GUM clinic, examination of the discharge under a microscope can give a provisional result so that treatment can be started earlier. The provisional result is confirmed by culture in the laboratory. In men a swab from the urethra or a urine sample is sent (preferably both). For women, diagnosis is usually made from the culture of a swab taken from the top of the vagina into a suitable transport medium. Urine samples do not give reliable results in women.

In other clinics, diagnosis is normally made by culture from swabs from the vagina or urethra. An incorrect diagnosis can be made from a cervical smear. The false positive rate (up to 30 out of 100 smears reported as having *Trichomonas vaginalis*) may cause psychological harm and unwarranted accusations of partner unfaithfulness. The diagnosis should always be confirmed by culture before treatment.

Gonorrhoea

This infection is caused by the bacteria *Neiserria gonorrhoea* (also known as gonococcus). About 10% of men and 50% of women can have the infection without any symptoms. In men complaints of dysuria (painful urination), discharge or epididymitis (painful swelling at the upper end of the testis) should raise your suspicions. Similarly in women, discharge, dysuria or abdominal pain can occur. The gonococcus infects mucous membranes so swabs need to be taken from the urethra or the endocervix (inner area of the cervix). Other sites (pharyngeal or rectal swabs) may be indicated by the sexual history.

Chlamydia

This is a common cause of infertility, ectopic pregnancy and chronic pelvic infection or pain. Men may have urethritis, and ascending infection in men causes epididymitis (infection in the tubes above the testis) but evidence of male infertility is limited. Men may also have lower abdominal pain or arthritis. Women may have vaginal discharge, bleeding between periods or after sexual activity, an inflamed cervix (that may bleed on contact), urethritis, pelvic inflammatory disease and lower abdominal pain or arthritis. Maternal to infant transmission causes conjunctivitis and pneumonitis in the newborn. It may occur together with other STIs and may help in the transmission and acquisition of HIV infection.

Non-specific urethritis

This is defined as an infection of the urethra not caused by gonorrhoea. It is common in young men. Up to 40% of episodes of urethritis are in fact caused by chlamydia. Bacteria called *Mycoplasma genitalium* and *Ureaplasma urealyticum* are commonest amongst the other causative organisms. The diagnosis is mainly made by a combination of symptoms of painful urination and the presence of pus cells — more than five per high power field ($\times 400$) seen under the microscope when the urethral swab is spread onto a slide.

Herpes simplex

Although a less significant infection than other genital infections in terms of numbers, herpes infections cause severe distress. Both the common infection seen on the face (type 1 virus) and the genital infection (type 2) can occur on the genitals. The first attack is often extremely painful, sometimes causing retention of urine (inability to pass urine) because of the severe pain as urine passes over the lesions. Recurrent attacks prevent sexual enjoyment and adversely affect the quality of life permanently, especially if recurrences are frequent.

Human papilloma virus

First-ever presentation of genital warts is rising, with a significant rise in the 16–19 year old age group. HPV infection is common amongst sexually active young people, whether or not visible warts are present. Genital warts are usually spread sexually, so their presence should prompt a search for other infections.

Human immunodeficiency virus

HIV means human immunodeficiency virus; AIDS means acquired immune deficiency syndrome.

HIV is present in blood, semen and vaginal fluids of people who are infected. People infected with HIV look and feel healthy most of the time. The virus slowly damages the immune system so that those infected are less able to resist and recover from other infections. Eventually that person will get infections or cancers that do not usually affect people who have healthy immune systems. When one or more of these illnesses occurs, people are defined as having AIDS.

Investigation

The HIV test looks for HIV antibodies in the blood, and it normally takes three months for antibodies to develop. If someone goes for an HIV test soon after possible infection, antibodies may not have had time to develop. The test result may be inaccurate and they will need to be tested again three months after possible infection to get a definite result.

Anyone in the UK can have a free HIV test. The test is available from any GUM clinic and the GP isn't informed that the patient has had a test, or of the result, without the patient's consent. More general practices are offering the HIV test and if health professionals work in an area with a higher prevalence rate, they need to think how best to arrange the procedures for testing. A counsellor, doctor or nurse should explain the test procedure and discuss possible results. It normally takes a week for the test result to return from the laboratory.

Implications of having an HIV test

Having a test may make it more difficult or more expensive to obtain life insurance or loans, such as mortgages backed by life insurance. It may also prevent travel or emigration to certain countries that require a declaration of freedom of infection from HIV before entry. Patients need to be told how requests for tests and their results will be stored in a way that makes inadvertent disclosure as unlikely as possible. Informed consent should always be obtained before disclosure to a third party. However, treatments can extend and improve the quality of life and reduce transmission from mothers to babies. Having a positive result commonly changes people's sexual behaviour to low-risk activities. Overall, for individuals at risk, the potential benefits of having an HIV test outweigh the disadvantages.

If the test is negative, the patient is unlikely to be infected unless infection occurred within the last three months. If the test is positive, the virus will probably remain in the body for the rest of that person's life. The patient is infectious to others and needs to consider preventing spread of the infection to others by avoiding unsafe sexual activities, sharing needles or syringes, or blood donation. Women should discuss their special requirements if having a baby (as the virus can be passed onto the baby at birth and by breast-feeding). HIV is *not* spread by ordinary social contact, sharing eating utensils, hugging or shaking hands. If there is a risk of having a positive result, the patient might want to consider returning for the result with a friend or other supporter, and not planning any other commitments afterwards for a while so that there is time to come to terms with the result. The patient needs to think about how to tell other people and who to tell. Some women have found that they are at increased risk of abuse after receiving a positive test result and disclosing this to a partner. Patients need access to the many support services that exist for HIV people, but may find it difficult to use these services when they are first informed about the result. It is common for people to deny the reality of any bad news initially.

In 2001, the Anonymous Prevalence Study[6] showed a rise in HIV prevalence in heterosexual GUM clinic attendees. The prevalence of HIV infection in pregnant women also continued to rise in England. HIV transmission among homosexual and bisexual men is continuing at a high rate in London (one in seven homosexual and bisexual men attending GUM clinics in London and one in 43 elsewhere were infected with HIV).

The prevalence of HIV is far higher in GUM clinic attendees born abroad, particularly in male and female heterosexuals born in sub-Saharan Africa. Of HIV-infected women giving birth in the UK in 2001, 70% lived in London and 77% were born in sub-Saharan Africa.[6]

A significant increase in previously undiagnosed HIV prevalence has been observed in heterosexual women. Between 1996 and 2001, after adjustment for age and centre effects, the prevalence of previously undiagnosed HIV infection in heterosexual women attending GUM clinics in London increased at an average annual rate of 3.7%.[6]

In 2001, there were an estimated 561 births to HIV-infected women in the UK, compared to 298 in 1997. This would have resulted in about 149 HIV-infected infants in 2001 if none of these maternal infections had been diagnosed, assuming a mother-to-infant transmission rate of about 25% in the absence of interventions. However, given the observed proportion of maternal infections diagnosed before delivery, and assuming that about 2% of infants will acquire HIV even if the maternal infection is diagnosed prior to delivery, it is estimated that some 49 infants were infected with HIV in 2001. These estimates indicate that although the number of births to HIV-infected women in the UK has risen, the estimated proportion of infants born to these women who are themselves infected has declined from about 19% in 1997 to about 9% in 2001.[6]

Although the uptake of voluntary confidential testing continues to improve in all groups of people attending GUM clinics both in and outside London, a significant number of HIV-infected people still remain undiagnosed after the clinic visit because of refusal to be tested. In 2001, substantial improvements in the detection of HIV infections in pregnant women were seen in England and Scotland, and around 100 infections in newborn infants were prevented because of greater willingness of women to be tested and the greater availability of testing. There was considerable variation between health authorities, however, in the antenatal HIV infection diagnosis rate (see Chapter 5).

At the end of 2001 an estimated 41 200 adults aged 16 years and over were living with HIV in the UK, 12 900 (31%) of whom were unaware of their infection, having been identified by anonymous testing. An estimated 19 500 adults who had acquired their infection through heterosexual sex were living in the UK in 2001, and 8300 (43%) of these were unaware of their infection. The rest had acquired their infection through sex with other men or from drug use. This has considerable implications for primary care and for improvements in the accessibility and normality of providing testing within primary care.

If you are to provide testing within general practice or in FP clinics, you should be up to date with the methods of testing and how long it takes for the antibodies to be present in the blood (usually about 12 weeks but some strains of HIV are different). You should be able to discuss with the patient the implications of being tested, how to reduce the risks of acquiring HIV and what to do if the test is positive. There is a useful advice document called *Take the HIV Test*[7] which would help in preparing yourself before providing this service. It offers advice to health professionals, especially doctors and midwives, on how to provide HIV testing straightforwardly and concisely. It reflects a growing view among health professionals that HIV testing should be a normal investigation alongside other diagnostic tests and procedures. People with HIV may assume that they have been given a clean bill of health, when in reality they have simply not been tested. Health professionals should offer the test, or advise where it can be done, so that people understand it will *not* be done unless they specifically agree. Include advice on prevention from infection in any discussion about HIV testing.

Rapid testing for HIV
The Food and Drug Administration in the USA has approved a rapid HIV test that can give a result within an hour.[8] The ability to give rapid results would reduce the difficulties of providing test results after a delay of a week. A proportion of patients do not return for their results and some of these have given no consent or information that would enable clinics to trace them. A rapid result would also be much more comfortable for patients. Most people would rather wait an hour than a week in anxious anticipation. Both those with negative and positive HIV test results who have put themselves at risk because of their activities need advice on how to change their behaviour, but those with positive results need more than this. The introduction of rapid testing would reduce the amount of counselling required so as to target it more extensively to those with positive results.

Anonymous testing for prevalence[6]
Most of the surveys test for HIV in blood samples left over after completion of routine clinical tests. The survey of GUM clinic attendees uses residual blood taken for syphilis serology. Surveys of pregnant women attending antenatal and termination clinics use samples taken for rubella serology and blood grouping respectively. The dried blood spot survey uses blood taken from

newborn infants for routine metabolic screening to test for maternal antibodies to HIV. Samples from people who objected to their blood being tested were not examined.

In purchasing primary care, as well as for prison and other health services, the Department of Health[6] suggests that primary care organisations should give appropriate priority to:

- HIV prevention activity and local needs assessment for:
  - homosexual and bisexual men
  - people from sub-Saharan African countries with high HIV prevalence
  - heterosexuals at behavioural risk of acquiring STIs
  - needle exchange and other harm minimisation services for injecting drug users (and users likely to progress to injecting)
  - people who are HIV-positive
- developing services for the increasing number of African men and women
- continue improving and monitoring the uptake of HIV testing by pregnant women
- reducing the transmission of HIV and other STIs in accordance with good practice as set out in the *National Strategy for Sexual Health and HIV: implementation action plan*[9]
- reducing the prevalence of undiagnosed HIV by working towards the national standard for GUM services to offer an HIV test to all clinic attendees on their first screening for STIs, and subsequently according to risk.

Other conditions found on investigation for STIs

Thrush (also known as Moniliasis or Candidiasis)

This is very common and *not* classified as a STI. It is caused by a fungal infection called *Candida albicans*. The first attack may be extremely uncomfortable with the itching, swelling, soreness and discharge causing considerable distress. Although often described as typically presenting with white 'cottage cheese' – like patches over bright red areas of the vulva or the vaginal walls, this appearance is more frequent in pregnancy. The discharge may be very variable and the vulva may have little splits or be red and shiny from frequent scratching. Most women complain mainly of itching and soreness, a rapid onset often in the pre-menstrual week and painful urination and/or sexual intercourse.

Recurrent thrush is defined as at least four symptomatic episodes within 12 months, proven as thrush by taking swabs. Only 5% of women with thrush have recurrent attacks. Current research suggests that women who have recurrent attacks are reacting in the same way to *Candida* as those with hay fever to pollens, i.e. they are producing an allergic reaction to the presence of *Candida* spores and hyphae on the vulval or vaginal mucosa.

Triggers for attacks of thrush are taking antibiotics, nylon or tight-fitting clothes, hygiene practices such as using soap, skin washes, bubble bath etc. to wash out the vagina, or using antiseptics in the vagina. Other conditions that increase the risk of thrush are pregnancy, high-dosage COCs (standard 20 or 30 microgram pills are *not* associated with an increased risk), diabetes mellitus, immune suppression, genital skin conditions (e.g. eczema or psoriasis) and sexual intercourse without a condom. All of these tend to decrease the level of acidity in the vagina and increase the risk of symptoms.

Men rarely have thrush as their genitals are kept much cooler. It may be more likely to develop under the foreskin if this is not kept clean and dry. It can be caught from a partner occasionally and is more likely to develop in damp, warm conditions, for example if the man has been sitting around in wet swimming trunks by a warm swimming pool. The appearance is similar to the vulva, with red shiny skin and sometimes small splits. Thrush is much more likely when resistance is lowered in diabetes, leukaemia or HIV infection. Frequent or severe symptoms should prompt a search for underlying conditions.

Bacterial vaginosis

This may be even more common than thrush. It is due to the overgrowth of predominately anaerobic bacteria (i.e. bacteria that prefer a lack of oxygen) that are normally present in only small numbers in the healthy vagina. They produce a fishy or ammonia smell in alkaline conditions so the condition may be worse after intercourse or just after the menstrual period has finished.

BV is a nuisance because of the smell and can put people off sexual intercourse. It usually only causes concern to health professionals if any surgical treatment is needed (as it may increase the risk of post-operative infection) or in pregnancy.

Making the diagnosis

Examination of the appearance of the genitals can be characteristic. More often there are no changes to be seen at all. Viral warts can be flat-topped, like miniature cauliflowers or filiform like a sea anemone. You may see a discharge of various colours. White and milky is usually thrush and in pregnancy may resemble cottage cheese. A grey and runny discharge is usually BV, especially if it smells fishy or ammoniacal. A green and frothy discharge may be TV.

Sometimes ulcers, or a rash, are seen. Occasionally you may be lucky enough to see pubic lice scuttling amongst the hairs with little flecks of bloodstaining on the underwear.

Tests

In men, plastic loops (these are very thin and are designed to slide easily into the urethra) are used to take samples of discharge from the urethra (the tube from the bladder to the outside), or swabs (cotton wool wrapped onto the end of a stick of wood, plastic or metal) are used to collect material from skin sores. The swabs are placed in a culture medium to keep the infective material alive until it can be examined in the laboratory.

In women, similar types of swabs are used to take samples of discharge from the upper vagina behind the cervix (neck of the uterus), from the cervix and from the urethra.

In both men and women, urine samples are taken for examination. Other body areas may be swabbed as indicated by the sexual history. The sexual history is necessary both to establish the level of risk of a STI and the type of sexual activity so that the correct body sites can be examined. Also in both men and women, blood tests are used for identifying infection with hepatitis, HIV or syphilis.

The sexual history will help to establish the level of risk and what tests should **2** be taken. Take swabs from the mouth, rectum and other superficial sites as indicated by the history. You may want to refer people to the GUM clinic where all the tests can be done and examined promptly. In women, you may be providing testing as part of your service. Ensure that:

- you can transport the samples to the laboratory with the minimum of delay
- the woman is clear about what tests are being done
- you have informed consent
- you know how the individual will be contacted with the results
- you both know what will need to happen if any are positive.

Discuss confidentiality when completing the laboratory request form. If the patient requests, use a patient number or pseudonym on the request form and sample containers (make sure you record the patient's identification details somewhere safe for your own peace of mind). Give as much clinical detail as you can to assist the laboratory in the interpretation of the results.

Urine testing

Send the first passed part of the urine for chlamydia, TV and non-specific urethritis testing, depending on what tests are available in the local laboratory. If the patient has passed urine within half to one hour of this sample, a false negative may be given as the urine may have washed away the bacteria. The mid-stream part of the urine (MSU) is used to diagnose urinary tract infections. A report on a MSU stating that white blood cells (indicating inflammation) are present, but with no growth of bacteria, suggests a chlamydia infection and should prompt you to do further tests if you did not do so at the time.

Swabs

For gonococcus and other bacterial infections, use a wooden or plastic-shafted swab to take material (from the urethra in men and the cervix in women) into charcoal medium.

For chlamydia testing of the urethra in both men and women, use a thin wire swab and place in the chlamydia testing pack.

In women, know which testing procedure your microbiology department uses. If it is enzyme immuno-assay (EIA) then an endocervical swab for women is the most effective, and if the urethral swab is sent as well this will increase your detection rate. Use the special chlamydial testing kit supplied by your laboratory for taking samples from the cervix. You must follow the instructions that come with the pack from the laboratory as each type of pack has different instructions. Some are very clear and state that the cleaning swab (the large bulbous swab of the two) must not be used as the swab for chlamydia. First clean any mucus off the cervix with the cleaning swab and then use the chlamydia swab (the metal or plastic-handled, thin, flat-ended swab). Rotate it for a minimum of 30 seconds in the cervix. Take cells from the transitional zone (the junction between the outer cells of the cervix and the inner ones lining the cervical canal). Remove the swab from the vagina and place it in the container supplied in accordance with the instructions.

To identify candida, BV and TV in women, a high vaginal swab can be taken from the top of the vagina. This is placed in Stuart's medium.

Staff in clinics and some GP surgeries can take viral swabs for herpes simplex from any small ulcers.

Blood tests

Take the history first. It is pointless taking a test for HIV or syphilis for someone recently exposed. The tests can take up to three months to become positive. Hepatitis A is usually diagnosed in the acute phase by specific immunoglobulin (IgM) antibodies, as these only persist for a short time.

Take advice from the local laboratory about the tests for hepatitis B, C, D and E, which are diagnosed by the various antibodies present at different stages of infection.

Chlamydia testing

The usually recommended test for chlamydia is the nucleic acid amplification **3**
test (NAAT) on urine (or on penile or vaginal discharge), but this may not be
available in your area. Testing the urine (the whole specimen, not a mid-stream
specimen) is much more acceptable than a swab from the urethra or cervix,
especially if a genital examination is not needed for other reasons.

Enzyme-immune antibody (EIA) tests on cervical or penile swabs may be the
only ones available but are less specific and sensitive. That is, the test may give
more false negative or false positive results (see Chapter 5). Chlamydia culture
does not give the best result from the point of view of sensitivity, having only
about a 60–70% sensitivity. However, culture is highly specific and is preferred
for tests required for legal purposes (e.g. after rape) as NAATs may sometimes
be falsely positive. Swabs with plastic or metal shafts are used as wooden shafts
are toxic to chlamydia. Taking swabs from other sites (e.g. the rectum or back of
the mouth) in either men or women depends on the sexual history obtained.

Human papilloma virus

Some HPVs (types 16, 18, 31, 33 and 35) – not usually the ones presenting as
visible warts – are associated with the development of cervical cancer. Yearly
cervical screening for five years is normally suggested if wart virus is found on
the cervix when cervical screening is done. Determining the type of HPV
present is still a research technique at present. Investigations are underway to
see if typing the virus can be used to distinguish between those people who
require more frequent follow-up and those whose infection is likely to be
transient and not associated with a greater risk of cervical cancer.

Vaccines are on trial for types 16 and 18 (the commonest ones associated
with cervical cancer). See Chapter 5 for more information on cervical cancer
screening.

Best practice in treatment

Sexual partners should be treated at the same time as the person with the STI **1**
(if possible) and abstinence from sexual intercourse is advised until treatment of
all partners is completed. Condom use reduces the risk of infection but abstinence is better. If one infection is found, screening for other infections must
also be arranged. Screening and tracing of sexual contacts is best done by the
GUM clinic.

Always check recent guidelines for treatment unless you are sure of the correct **2**
medication and dose. Good sources of advice are listed at the end of this section
(p. 185). You may have specific guidelines on treatment in your area and they

may have been drawn up because some infections have become resistant to commonly used treatments. People can obtain treatment from GUM clinics free from prescription charges, or from their general practice surgery with the usual prescription charges. Some sexual health and FP clinics have a budget to give treatment, but it is more usual for them to write to the GP to ask them to prescribe.

Trichomoniasis

Usually give metronidazole tablets either as a single dose of 2 g or as a five-day course of 400 mg twice a day.[4] It is important the full course is completed or the infection may return. Advise that alcohol is avoided while on the tablets or vomiting may occur.

Gonorrhoea

Referral to a GUM clinic for full STI screening, contact tracing and advice on current antibiotic sensitivities is best practice. *Neiserria gonorrhoea* has become resistant to commonly used antibiotics in some areas. It is essential that female contacts are traced and treated as long-term adverse effects from pelvic infection can occur even in women without any complaints.

Chlamydia

In uncomplicated infections of the lower genital tract (urethra and/or cervix), men and non-pregnant women are usually given azithromycin 1 g as a single dose, doxycycline 100 mg twice daily for seven days, or oxytetracycline 250 mg four times daily for seven days. Pregnant women are advised to have azithromycin 1 g as a single dose, erythromycin 500 mg four times a day for seven days, or amoxicillin 500 mg three times daily for seven days.[4] If there has been spread of the infection from the lower genital tract, seek specialist advice. Screening for other infections and treatment of all sexual contacts is best done by the GUM clinic.

Non-specific urethritis

The partner(s) should be treated to prevent recurrence. Treatment is as for chlamydia.

Herpes simplex

Sitting in a warm bath with about a cupful of salt in it makes passing urine much more comfortable. Oral antiviral treatment reduces the duration of symptoms, lesions and viral shedding. Research reports that daily treatment reduces recurrences and may improve the quality of life. There is some evidence that condom use reduces rates of transmission.

HPV

Podophyllin paint is usually used first. This is very irritating and should be washed off three to four hours after its application. It is not suitable for self-application as it is easy to overtreat in the hope of a speedy cure and have nasty burns, or even peripheral neuropathy (damage to nerves), hypokalaemia (low potassium levels that can be toxic to the heart) or coma after applying large quantities.

    Podophyllotoxin 0.5% has less severe side-effects and can be applied at home if the sufferer can accurately localise the warts (easier with penile warts than those in other positions!). Trichloracetic acid, electrocautery (heat treatment) or cryotherapy (freezing) are also used for larger or more resistant warts.[4]

The effects of treatment are difficult to evaluate because of natural regression **3** (about 30%) and also recurrences after treatment. There is no evidence yet that treatment of external warts reduces the risk of infecting others. Using a condom has not been adequately evaluated, but seems a sensible precaution.[4]

HIV

Evidence suggests that combination treatment with several drugs is more **2** successful in preventing resistance to medication. Treatment of other STIs can reduce the likelihood of acquiring HIV. Seek specialist advice.

    There is no cure for HIV infection, but there are a number of drugs that can help prevent someone who is HIV-positive from becoming ill. In the UK, an HIV-positive person can get free treatment for HIV. Highly active antiretroviral treatment (HAART) has resulted in great improvements in the health status of many individuals with HIV. They do seem to have side-effects (in common with most effective treatments!) and are associated with premature atherosclerosis (narrowing of the arteries with difficulties in maintaining the coronary and peripheral circulation).

Treatment consists of taking several drugs every day (combination therapy) for life. If the drugs are not taken correctly, the treatment will stop being so effective and the person may become ill. Taking combination therapy increases the life expectancy of a person who is HIV-positive by several years.

Drug treatment can also help to prevent an HIV-positive pregnant woman passing on the infection to her unborn child. Testing during the first 12 weeks of pregnancy and starting treatment then if required reduces the risk of transmission of infection to the baby from an estimated 25% to about 2%.

Thrush

Care of the vulval skin and vagina should include:

- keep dry and cool
- have showers not baths
- no douching (washing out the vagina)
- avoid perfumes, soap, detergents, antiseptics and deodorants (preparations 'balanced' for the skin are for pH 7.4, not the pH 4.6 of the vagina)
- use aqueous cream instead of soap.

Anti-fungal therapy usually clears the thrush – resistance is very rare. Recurrent attacks may need three to six months continuous or intermittent therapy (dependent on the cause) and some people need bigger doses as with any medication. Clotrimazole, econazole, ketoconazole, miconazole and isoconazole are available as cream or pessaries. Both the vagina and the vulva need treatment. The pessaries to treat the vagina are more expensive over the counter than a prescription charge currently in the UK, but the cream is not. Women may prefer just to have a prescription for the pessaries and buy the cream themselves. Short courses are easier to finish. Nystatin pessaries and cream are less effective and require a 14-day course. Oral treatment with fluconazole (one 150 mg tablet) or itraconazole (200 mg repeated once after eight hours) is popular, especially if the vulva is very inflamed. The oral treatment should be avoided in pregnancy, is more expensive and does not have a higher cure rate.

Bacterial vaginosis

This can resolve spontaneously. Avoiding hygiene practices that disturb the vaginal bacteria helps to prevent it. Causes of alteration of vaginal bacteria include blood in the vagina from menstrual loss or after delivery, a foreign body such as a tampon or pessary, ejaculate after intercourse or other infections. Many women improve with simple measures by correcting the alteration of the vaginal flora, particularly by preventing the entry of detergents, soaps and other 'skin-friendly' preparations made to keep the pH at 7.4, not that of the more acid vagina.

Oral treatment is metronidazole 2 g as one dose or 400 mg twice daily for five to seven days; vaginal treatment is metronidazole gel 0.75% for five days or clindamycin cream 2% for seven days (the clindamycin cream can cause condom weakening).

Do not treat the partner. There is no evidence for a 'rectal reservoir' of infection. After antibiotic treatment many people will have further evidence of BV — about six in ten people in the next three months.

The barriers to effective treatment and diagnosis

The main obstacles are the lack of knowledge about STIs and that so often they do not give any symptoms or signs, so people do not know they have an infection. People tend to rate themselves as 'clean' and think that only people who 'sleep around' get STIs. It is difficult to obtain good quality diagnosis and treatment because of lack of easy access to GUM clinics and the perception that going to a clinic is stigmatising or exposing an individual to blame. Some people will not attend a local clinic for fear of being identified, but access to more distant clinics may be even more difficult.

People do not do what health professionals tell them to do unless they understand and accept the need to do so. Concordance is a negotiated agreement on treatment between the patient and the healthcare professional that allows patients to take informed decisions on the degree of risk or suffering that they themselves wish to undertake or follow. In contrast, 'compliance' with treatment or lifestyle changes implies that the patient follows instructions from health professionals to a greater or lesser degree.[10]

The attitudes of health professionals and others in contact with sexually active people can make the difference between them feeling able to seek help or advice and accepting the need for changes in sexual behaviour, or rejecting the advice and continuing to put themselves and others at risk.

Assessing someone's readiness to make changes is a skill to be learned. People pass through the stages of:

- being happy with their present state or behaviour
- acknowledging that there is a problem

- accepting that they need to change
- changing
- maintaining the change, or reverting to previous habits.

Service provision within traditional settings can be improved. Recommendations include linking services and delivering care without personal judgement. The report for the Department of Health by the Health Education Authority *Reducing the Rate of Teenage Conceptions*[11] singles out vulnerable young people as being 'hard to reach'. A paper linking the provision of emergency contraception in general practice and termination of pregnancy[12] showed that teenagers were attending general practices for contraception, but not necessarily continuing to take precautions against the sexual health risks that they were taking. **3**

Some young people may regard all older people or professionals as imposing their own decisions without consultation and discussion. They often hold their peers in much higher regard. Consider how this could be used to inform and educate young people of the need for safer sexual practices.

Other barriers include the traditionally poor provision for sexual health services. Until recently most GUM clinics were hidden away from public view and in Dickensian buildings with inadequate facilities. There are still too few clinics, too few health professionals staffing them, with restricted opening hours and little provision for rapid, open access. Access is restricted if someone has to wait for two weeks for an appointment, or has to take time off from work to attend. The potential for not attending is increased and with it the chances of spread of STIs to others. Provision outside GUM clinics is not always of a high standard because of lack of resources, staff and knowledge. There is sometimes an unwillingness to provide for this area as STIs are often viewed as 'self-imposed illness' and that which should be avoided by behavioural changes, rather than accepting the world as it is and coping with the results. Large-scale behavioural change cannot be achieved by medical intervention alone.

How can further infection be prevented?

Effective diagnosis and treatment, with treatment of *all* sexual contacts, can prevent further spread of infection. Then advise changes in sexual behaviour to avoid or minimise the risk in future. Monogamous monogamy (each in a partnership only ever having sex with each other) is ideal. Any change in partner should prompt precautions such as the use of a condom to reduce the risk. **1**

Helping people to understand the risks of STIs and how they can control them for themselves is an important part of treatment. Without it, clients can return reinfected and with the potential of having infected others. **2**

Concealment of sexual activity, or the need to do so because of the fear of dis- **3**
approval or sanctions by partners, social grouping or religious establishments,
can be a powerful motivation to prevent effective contact tracing and treatment. Awareness of the difficulties that some cultures and religions impose can
make all the difference between ineffective or successful treatment and the prevention of further infection.

Further learning

You may want to consult reference documents for the latest on management **3**
and treatment of STIs. The following publications will give you a good start:

> *Clinical Evidence* (latest issue) – editorial team and advisors. BMJ Publishing
> Group, London. Also at http://www.clinicalevidence.com.
> *British National Formulary* (latest issue) – Joint Formulary Committee. British
> Medical Association and Royal Pharmaceutical Society of Great Britain,
> London. Also at http://www.bnf.org.
> *Guidelines: summarising clinical guidelines for primary care* (latest issue) – repre-
> sentatives of professional bodies and organisations producing guidelines.
> Medendium Group Publishing Ltd, Berkhamstead. Also at http://www.
> eguidelines.co.uk. This gives you the source for the full guidelines for any
> particular condition.

Look in the Appendix for other sources of information.

References

1 Wakley G and Chambers R (2001) *Sexual Health Matters in Primary Care.* Radcliffe
  Medical Press, Oxford.
2 British Medical Association (2002) *Sexually Transmitted Infections.* British Medical
  Association, London.
3 Department of Health (2001) *National Strategy for Sexual Health and HIV.* Department of Health, London. Also on www.doh.gov.uk/nshs.
4 Jones G (ed) (2003) *Clinical Evidence* **8**. BMJ Publishing Group, London.
5 Harvey J, Webb A and Mallinson H (2000) Chlamydia trachomatis screening in
  young people in Merseyside. *British Journal of Family Planning* **26**: 199–201.
6 Department of Health (2002) *Prevalence of Hepatitis and HIV in the United Kingdom:
  annual report of the Unlinked Anonymous Prevalence Monitoring Programme.* Department of Health, London.

7 Members of the BMA Foundation for AIDS (2002) *Take the HIV Test.* Medical Foundation for AIDS and Sexual Health, BMA House, Tavistock Square, London WC1H 9JP. Website: http://www.medfash.org.uk.

8 Rotheram-Borus MJ and Etzel MA (2000) Effective detection of HIV. *Journal of AIDS* **25** (2): 105–14.

9 Department of Health (2002) *The National Strategy for Sexual Health and HIV: implementation action plan.* Department of Health, London.

10 Royal Pharmaceutical Society of Great Britain (1997) *From Compliance to Concordance: towards shared goals in medicine taking.* Royal Pharmaceutical Society of Great Britain, London.

11 Meyrick J and Swann C (1998) *Reducing the Rate of Teenage Conceptions: an overview of the effectiveness of interventions and programmes aimed at reducing unintended conceptions in young people.* Health Education Authority, London.

12 Churchill D, Allen J, Pringle M *et al.* (2000) Consultation patterns and provision of contraception in general practice before teenage pregnancy: case–control study. *British Medical Journal* **321**: 486–9.

8

More about men

Gender differences

What are the inequalities between women's and men's health?

For the population in the UK healthy life expectancy increased only slightly **1** between 1990 and 1999, from 66.1 to 66.6 years for men and from 68.3 to 68.9 years for women. Overall life expectancy has increased more than healthy life expectancy, so life expectancy whilst in poorer health has increased (75.1 years for men, 80.0 years for women).[1]

The White Paper *Saving Lives – Our Healthier Nation*[2] highlights the already wide health gap in the main disease groups, yet policy makers are still concentrating on women's health issues.

Men are much less likely than women to visit the doctor when they feel ill.[3] They are traditionally brought up to be brave and tough, to shrug off pain from any scrapes, subscribing to the notion that if a male shows concern for his health he appears to be less masculine. Then in adulthood the pressures of life, work and family mean that men tend to put off visiting the doctor when they are ill and may neglect their health, taking their good health for granted.

Men could benefit from equivalent health checks to those that women have been taking advantage of for some time. Most general practices provide some form of male health clinics or checks, including measuring blood pressure and cholesterol levels. Information and advice is available on giving up smoking, exercise, healthy eating, alcohol consumption and coping with stress for both men and women.

Most men do not take advantage of the same social support networks that **2** women access, such as sharing their problems with friends and family. Often it is the man's partner who notices changes in his health and encourages a visit to the doctor or practice nurse.

Possible inequalities in men and women's sexual health

Statistics about STIs published by the Public Health Laboratory Service (PHLS) **2** since 1995[4] show that there are inequalities between the sexes for uncomplicated gonorrhoea and syphilis.

Uncomplicated gonorrhoea

In 2001 the numbers diagnosed in GUM clinics in England with uncomplicated gonorrhoea were 63 men per 100 000 compared to 26 women in 100 000. Since 1995, diagnosis of uncomplicated gonorrhoea in males has increased by 130% in heterosexually acquired, and by 160% in homosexually acquired, infections.

These figures might be explained by some infections being acquired through men having sex with men. Also men are more likely to be symptomatic than women, and therefore more likely to access a sexual health service. Women are more likely to attend general practice and might not appear in the statistics.

Syphilis

Recent statistics show a marked increase in syphilis in males during the 1990s. Although the figures for syphilis in England are lower than the rates for other STIs, they have increased sharply since 1998 from 0.3 to 2.4 men per 100 000. The PHLS explains that these sharp increases are accounted for by outbreaks occurring in Bristol, Manchester, Brighton, Cambridgeshire and London, mainly among men who have sex with men.

Chlamydia

The figures for uncomplicated genital chlamydia are higher in females than males − 151 women per 100 000 compared to 118 men per 100 000 in 2001.[4] There are more opportunities for women to be referred to a GUM clinic for chlamydia testing than men. For example, chlamydia could be picked up at cervical screening, before an IUD insertion or before a termination of pregnancy. At present, men usually only have the opportunity for a chlamydia test when they present at a GUM clinic and have full STI screening.

Herpes

In 2001, the rates of HSV infection (first attack) were lower in men than women, occurring in 91 men per 100 000 aged 20–24 years compared with 193 women per 100 000 of the same age group in England, Wales and Northern Ireland.[4] It is unclear why the diagnosis of herpes is higher in women than men but may reflect men's reluctance to access health services.

Historically, the needs of men have not been considered separately from those of women when sexual health services have been planned, although they make up a significant proportion of the groups which have been identified as having specific needs, i.e. young people, black and ethnic minorities, unemployed, those suffering mental illness and gay and bisexual groups. There is a great deal of scope for policy makers to improve men's opportunities to achieve good health. For instance, the cost-effectiveness of rolling out national screening programmes for prostate cancer is currently being researched (see Chapter 5) and could be considered in the future in much the same way as cervical and breast cancer screening is currently in place for women.[3]

3

Factors contributing to male sexual ill health

Basic hygiene rules for males

Many men do not realise that it is important for them to wash around their genitals, anus and pubic hair every day, and, if they have not been circumcised, to ensure that the foreskin of the penis is rolled back and thoroughly cleaned underneath. This helps to prevent infection and reduce the risk of developing penile cancer. A health professional may need to tell male patients tactfully about washing.

1

If the foreskin is not cleaned underneath on a regular basis, a minor infection may cause the tip of the penis to become swollen and tender, tightening the foreskin. The foreskin will not then be able to be pulled back all the way up the shaft of the penis. This condition is called phimosis and can be treated with antibiotics and an improved hygiene regime.

No attempt should be made to force the foreskin back, but a gradual process of pulling it back slightly, a bit further every day, may be required until the foreskin is fully retracted. Application of steroid creams may help. It is not always possible to achieve a full retraction and referral to a urologist in hospital may be required for surgical intervention – a small snip in the foreskin or a full circumcision.

Circumcision

Circumcision is the complete surgical removal of the foreskin. This operation is normally performed for religious reasons, for example Muslim and Jewish boys are normally circumcised in childhood. It is occasionally necessary as a treatment for phimosis (see above).

Working with chemicals

Males often work with materials that contain carcinogenic elements, such as machine and motor oils and various chemicals. Other materials, such as plaster or mortar, contain irritants such as lime. It is very important therefore that men working with chemicals wash their hands *before and after* going to the toilet. Wearing protective gloves that are removed before passing urine will also protect the penis. Consider if the occupation of the man is relevant if he presents with a rash or sore on the penis or genital area. Sometimes men apply over-the-counter creams in an attempt to treat a suspected infection rather than consult a doctor or nurse. Medicinal creams or lotions should not be applied to the genital area unless specifically prescribed by a doctor or nurse, or after consultation with a pharmacist. They may complicate the diagnosis by altering the appearance of the rash or encourage infection by providing traces of cream in which bacteria can thrive.

If the man has detected a smell under his foreskin then washing with salt water morning and night for a few days may be all that is required to solve the problem. General practice health professionals or those at the local GUM clinic can investigate if washing regularly does not resolve the problem.

Salt-water bathing

This treatment is particularly useful during a herpes outbreak or during wart treatment and will encourage healing as well as preventing infection.

Encourage men suffering from warts or herpes to place a cupful of salt in the bath, or a tablespoon in a suitable container such as a large clean jam jar, and soak the penis for about five minutes. They should rinse off the salt solution in clean water and dry the penis with a towel. If there is broken skin they should not rub this area with a towel but dry with the *cool* setting of a hair-dryer, taking care not to burn the skin area.

Signs of infection

Not all infections will give symptoms but if any of the following are present   **1**
then they should be investigated at a GUM clinic, or by a GP or nurse:

- burning feeling or pain on passing urine
- feeling of wanting to pass urine often
- itching in the genital area
- pain in the genital area
- sore testicles
- a foul smell
- rash in the genital area
- lumps in the genital area
- sores/ulcers in the genital area
- discharge from the penis.

Any 'discharge' from the penis is abnormal and should be investigated. However, it is important to establish what a young man means when he complains   **2**
of a discharge. If his discharge only occurs during the night or when he wakes
up in the morning, the 'discharge' he is describing may be a 'wet dream' where
he has ejaculated semen in his sleep, and he can be reassured that this is
perfectly normal.

Unprotected sex

One of the main contributors to male sexual ill health is unprotected sex; that is,   **1**
sex without using a barrier such as a condom. Some STIs have no symptoms and
cause significant damage as they go undetected for long periods of time. For
example, hepatitis causes liver damage and syphilis causes heart or brain damage.

Infections can be passed to partners during oral and anal sex as well as vaginal
penetration. Barrier methods such as condoms should always be used for
any penetrative intercourse if there is any risk of infection – and a risk should be
assumed unless the sexual history of the partner is known with certainty. Due
to the frequency of STIs, especially amongst the under-25 year olds, couples
should assume that a partner might have an infection and take appropriate
precautions in order to protect not only themselves, but also future partners.
The couple could suspend the use of barrier protection when a monogamous
couple have both had a full screen for STIs (available at a GUM clinic) and their
tests are negative.

Some common infections such as genital warts and genital herpes have no cure but can be managed with treatment. Other infections such as HIV and some types of hepatitis are life threatening and the risk of transmission is considerably reduced by using a condom.

Avoiding unsafe sex with condom use

For persons whose sexual behaviours place them at risk for STIs, correct and consistent use of the male latex condom can reduce the risk of STI transmission. However, no protective method is 100% effective, and condom use cannot guarantee absolute protection against any STI. Condoms lubricated with spermicides are no more effective than other lubricated condoms in protecting against the transmission of HIV and other STIs. In order to achieve the protective effect of condoms, they must be used correctly and consistently. Incorrect use can lead to condom slippage or breakage, thus diminishing their protective effect. Inconsistent use can lead to STI transmission because transmission can occur with a single act of intercourse.

A Cochrane review indicates that consistent use of condoms results in 80% reduction in HIV incidence. Consistent use is defined as using a condom for all acts of penetrative vaginal intercourse. Since studies tended not to specify the type of condom that was used, the review might not apply only to male latex condoms but to male condoms made of other material such as polyurethane. Effectiveness of condoms at preventing transmission of infection is slightly lower than the effectiveness of condoms measured by fertility rates as the latter will be affected by the background fertility of the couple using condoms.[5]

There are two main ways that STIs can be transmitted:

1 body fluid spread: HIV, as well as gonorrhoea, chlamydia and TV, are spread when infected semen or vaginal fluids meet mucosal surfaces (e.g. the male urethra, the vagina or cervix).
2 direct skin, or direct mucosal, surface contact: genital ulcer diseases, genital herpes and syphilis, and HPV are spread by contact with infected skin or mucosal surfaces.

Laboratory studies demonstrate that latex condoms provide a complete barrier to particles the size of STI pathogens. So theoretically condoms can be expected to provide different levels of protection for various STIs, depending on differences in how the diseases are transmitted. Because condoms block the discharge of semen or protect the male urethra against exposure to vaginal secretions, a greater level of protection is provided for diseases spread by the body fluids. A lesser degree of protection is provided for skin-to-skin contact, or mucosal contact spread, because the condom may not cover these surfaces.

It is easier to measure the protective effects of condoms where one partner is known to have an infection and the other is known not be infected. Most of the studies on HIV prevention have been carried out in this way and show a reduction in the expected rates of transmission of HIV in those who used condoms compared with those who did not.

Other studies have tried to measure the protective effect of condoms by comparing rates of various STIs between condom users and non-users in real-life settings. This is difficult because these studies involve private behaviours that investigators cannot observe directly and the level of exposure to STIs among study participants is not known. As a result, observed measures of condom effectiveness in preventing other STIs are likely to be inaccurate. The results of these studies vary widely, ranging from ones demonstrating no effect to others showing low rates of STIs associated with condom use.[5]

Infections and infertility

A previous infection with any STI, e.g. chlamydia, NSU etc., can affect the fertility of men because of damage to the testis or collecting tubules.   **2**

Other causes of infertility

There are a number of factors that impact on the quality and quantity of sperm, thereby affecting fertility in males.[6] They include:

- increasing age
- smoking
- excess alcohol consumption
- occupation
- frequency of intercourse
- previous medical problems
- presence of an abnormality.

Types of infection that may cause infertility

Orchitis
This is an inflammation of the testes and is usually caused by a blood-borne   **3**
virus, commonly mumps. Atrophy of the testes may result and cause sterility.

The treatment depends on the nature of the causative agent (see below) but there is no current treatment for mumps.[7]

Epididymitis
This is an inflammation of the epididymis, the collection of tubules at the top of the testis. It can occur as a result of trauma, chemical irritation from urine reflux, or more commonly, by an ascending infection. If severe it can also affect the testis when it is known as epididymo-orchitis.

In young men, epididymo-orchitis tends to be associated with sexually transmissible pathogens, including *Chlamydia trachomatis* and *Neisseria gonorrhoea.*

In men who practise insertive anal intercourse, enteric organisms may cause epididymo-orchitis from the gut.

In older men and in men who have undergone urinary tract instrumentation or catheterisation, epididymo-orchitis is more often associated with urinary tract organisms.

If sexual acquisition is suspected, empirical treatment should commence prior to laboratory confirmation and should cover both chlamydia and gonorrhoea. Patients should be offered screening for other STIs.

Symptoms include testicular pain and tenderness, usually only on one side. There may be redness and/or oedema of the scrotum, associated urethritis, often painful urination or urethral discharge.

Rest, scrotal support and elevation, and appropriate analgesia should be advised. Non-steroidal anti-inflammatory medication may give some symptomatic relief. Treatment depends on the causative organism, usually after culture and sensitivity investigations (see Chapter 7 for treatment of chlamydia and gonorrhoea).[7,8]

In young men the diagnosis can be confused with torsion of the testis, when the testis becomes twisted and does not lie straight in the scrotum. Torsion *must* be considered and excluded in any young man presenting with pain in the testis. Torsion commonly presents with sudden onset of severe pain and no evidence of urethritis or urinary tract infection. Torsion is more likely in men under the age of 20 years.

Prostate problems

The three main conditions that can affect the prostate gland are:

1 prostatitis (inflammation of the prostate gland)
2 benign (non-cancerous) enlargement of the prostate gland known as benign prostatic hyperplasia
3 prostate cancer (see p. 198).

The most common symptom of all three of these conditions is difficulty in passing urine. This is due to the urethra, the tube that carries the urine from the bladder, becoming narrowed by the enlargement of the prostate tissue. Men usually present to, and are treated in, general practice.

Prostatitis

Acute bacterial prostatitis is an inflammation of all or part of the prostate gland.   **2** It usually becomes infected by direct spread from the urethra or bladder, occasionally from the rectum, or distant spread by the blood or lymphatic systems. The bacteria most commonly involved are:

- gut organisms: *Escherichia coli* or *Streptococcus faecalis*
- *Staphylococcus aureus*
- *Neisseria gonorrhoea*.

The patient usually has symptoms of general infection, for example fever, chills and muscle pain. Symptoms of local infection commonly include perineal pain and difficulty passing urine with urinary frequency and urgency. Occasionally, there may be haematuria (blood in the urine) or an abscess in the prostate, with pain on defaecation.

On rectal examination, the prostate is tender and swollen. Prostatic massage may cause pus to be exuded from the urethra.

Treatment is with oral antibiotics – for example, ciprofloxacin, trimethoprim or tetracycline – these may need to be continued for at least six weeks.[9] Drainage of an abscess may be needed and is done via the urethra with a rectoscope or through the perineum. Avoid catheter use or cystoscopy as these procedures may make the infection worse.

Chronic prostatic inflammation can result from inadequately treated acute prostatitis, or genito-urinary tuberculosis, but the cause is frequently unknown. Men usually complain of chronic, low-grade perineal pain, usually varying in severity and frequency. The pain may be made worse by sitting on a hard chair. Other features may include low back pain, which may extend down the leg, mild bouts of fever and dysuria.

In men with an infection, rectal examination usually reveals an enlarged, firm and irregular prostate and massage may exudes a purulent urethral discharge. As for any chronic infection, check for diabetes. Treatment is with the use of an appropriate antibiotic, generally a fluroquinolone, for a course of four to eight weeks.

Chronic pain without evidence of inflammation is more common. Symptoms can include suprapubic, scrotal, testicular, penile or lower back pain or discomfort, known as prostodynia, in the absence of inflammation in prostatic secretions. Treatment with long-term antibiotics and the addition of an alpha-blocker is usually advised.[9] You may need to seek an opinion from a urologist.

Benign prostatic hyperplasia

BPH is very common, affecting one in three men over 50 years old, and is caused by the prostate gland enlarging and partially obstructing the flow of urine down the urethra. Many men will accept the symptoms as part of ageing, whilst others will complain at an early stage usually of:

2

- difficulty in passing urine
- delay in starting to pass urine
- a poor stream of urine
- having to pass urine more often, especially at night
- a feeling that the bladder has not completely emptied.

Initial treatment for those with troublesome symptoms is medical, but surgical reduction of the hypertrophied prostatic tissue may be required.[9]

In patients with mild to moderate symptoms who do not want treatment then watchful waiting is sensible. If patients have more troublesome symptoms then medical treatment should be tried first.

3

Initial treatment is with alpha-adrenoceptor blockers, e.g. alfuzasin, tamsulosin or terazosin. These drugs block sympathetic activity and relax the smooth muscle component of prostatic obstruction. Indoram and doxazasin are also alpha-adrenoceptor blockers used for hypertensive treatment as well.

Finasteride is best used in patients with large prostates — in this patient group finasteride may reduce the risk of acute retention and the need for subsequent surgery. It blocks the formation of dihydrotestosterone, producing reduction of the hypertrophied prostatic tissue.

Surgical treatment is indicated if there are severe symptoms or complications of BPH such as retention of urine. The main surgical treatment in the UK is transurethral resection of the prostate (TURP). Very unfit patients may benefit temporarily from balloon dilatation.

Refer patients for a specialist opinion from a urologist if:

- they have severe symptoms, particularly if these have developed rapidly
- rectal examination suggests a hard craggy prostate
- there are complications such as recurrent urinary infections, haematuria, urinary retention, obstructive nephropathy or bladder stones
- the PSA is raised above the normal range for your laboratory
- medical treatment has not controlled the symptoms.

Male cancers

There are three cancers which affect men only:

1

- penile cancer
- prostate cancer
- testicular cancer.

Bladder cancer is more common in men than women.

Penile cancer

This is a very rare cancer and has a very good chance of complete recovery, if diagnosed early enough. However, most men only seek help one year after the initial lesion has appeared, reducing the effectiveness of treatment dramatically. It affects approximately one in 100 000 men per year in most developed countries. It has been less common in men who have been circumcised, but this is probably due to poor hygiene in uncircumcised men rather than to the operation itself. It accounts for less than 1% of adult malignancies in Europe and the USA.[9] Advise men with worries about changes in the appearance of the penis to consult their GP or attend the GUM clinic.

Men whose potential for developing this type of cancer is greater include those:

- over 40 years old
- who don't wash under the foreskin
- who have viral infections of the genitals such as certain HPVs.

Penile cancer most commonly arises under the foreskin on the glans of the penis (the end of the penis). Look for:

2

- a raw area
- a wart-like growth
- a red, velvety patch
- swollen lymph nodes in the inguinal region (a less common symptom).

Investigations

The only sure way to diagnose penile cancer is to take a very small sample (biopsy) of the suspected area. This can be done under a local anaesthetic in a

3

GUM clinic or hospital unit and need not require a stay in hospital. The biopsy specimen is examined in a hospital laboratory. If the biopsy removes the whole affected area then this might be the only treatment that is necessary. However, the laboratory report may indicate that further treatment is required, such as radiotherapy or laser treatment.

If a biopsy confirms penile cancer further tests may be required, such as a body scan, ultrasound and needle biopsies of the lymph glands to assess whether and to what extent the cancer has spread.

Prostate cancer

The prostate gland is a small, walnut-sized gland just below the bladder. It **1** produces a fluid which makes up part of the semen. It can be felt on a rectal examination. Symptoms of prostate cancer are very similar to those of benign prostatic hypertrophy and include:

- urinary frequency
- night-time frequency
- urgency of urination
- hesitation before being able to pass urine.

Complaints of pain, blood in the urine, hip or back pain and impotence occur late in the condition.

Men over the age of 50 years old are most at risk. Rates increase with age and prostate cancer is the second highest cause of cancer-related deaths in men, after lung cancer. However, due to its slow progression and early detection and treatment, many men die *with* it as opposed to dying *from* it.

Diagnosis and treatment

A PSA blood test will usually show very raised levels in most men with prostate **2** cancer (see Chapter 5 on screening). Levels over 10 ng/ml are usually due to cancer, but can be found in prostatitis or significant BPH. An examination of the prostate through the rectum may show enlargement, an unusual hardness or lumpiness of the prostate.

An ultrasound examination may be helpful in localising a cancer. Diagnosis is usually done using a fine-needle biopsy via the rectum by the urologist as a hospital outpatient.

Treatment depends on a number of different factors, such as the age and state of health of the sufferer and the extent of spread of the disease at diagnosis.[9] If the patient is elderly and the cancer has not spread, then regular monitoring may be all that is required as the progression of the disease may be very slow and aggressive treatment may be detrimental to the quality of life of the patient.

Further investigations and treatment

Treatments include: **3**

- radical prostatectomy that removes all of the prostate gland. Impotence is a common problem after this operation because of damage to the nerves, and about 40% of men have incontinence of urine
- radiotherapy that is usually undertaken guided by a computer-aided programme focusing the radiotherapy on the cancerous area. Impotence and incontinence are less likely after local radiotherapy
- brachytherapy, that involves placing radioactive seeds inside the prostate gland through a needle. The radioactivity gradually decays but has been shown to be an effective treatment for localised cancer and causes a lower rate of complications
- hormone therapy if the cancer has spread to other parts of the body as the disease is reliant on the hormone testosterone.

If a biopsy confirms prostate cancer, further tests may be required, such as a body scan, ultrasound and needle biopsies of the lymph glands to assess whether the cancer has spread. If the cancer is not localised to the prostate, chemotherapy or radiotherapy may be needed to treat secondary deposits in addition to hormone treatment.

Lumps in the scrotum

The scrotum is the sac that hangs behind and below the penis and contains the   **1**
testes, the male sexual glands. The scrotum's primary function is to maintain the testes at approximately 34°C, the temperature at which the testes most effectively produce sperm. One testis often hangs lower than the other and it is normal for men to have one that is bigger than the other, although they are usually of the same weight. Usually only one testis is affected by testicular cancer.

Self-examination is a useful way of checking that there has not been any change in either testis. It is done by feeling the testis between the thumb and the index and middle finger, then gently squeezing and checking for any lumps or thickening. A good time to do this is after a warm bath or shower, when the muscles of the scrotal sac are most relaxed. If it is done in front of a mirror the man can check for any change in appearance.

Men may notice a painless lump or a thickening in part of the testis, or may have an altered sensation of heaviness or dragging.

If any changes are found then this should be checked in a GUM clinic or by a GP. If a lump is thought to be in the testis an ultrasound should be arranged.

Most lumps are not due to cancer of the testis. Other conditions more frequently found in the scrotum are:

- a hernia – a loop of bowel protruding down into the scrotum
- a hydrocoele – a collection of sterile fluid in the cord attached to the testis
- a varicocoele – a collection of veins in similar position
- a cyst of the epididymis, the collecting tubules above and to the side of the testis.

Small lumps on the outside skin of the scrotum could be warts (see Chapter 7), but are often normal hair follicles or sweat glands that become more prominent in cold weather or when the penis is erect.

Who is at risk of testicular cancer?

All men can be at risk from testicular cancer, but there are some groups whose **1** potential for developing this type of cancer is greater:

- those aged between 15 and 50 years old, with the 20–34 year age group at the highest risk
- those with a close male relative (brother or father) with testicular cancer
- those with an undescended testis, which was not corrected in childhood
- those with a sedentary lifestyle.

Diagnosis and treatment

When a presumed diagnosis of testicular cancer has been made, the affected **2** testis will usually be removed under general anaesthetic and sent for histological examination. It may be possible for the man to have an artificial implant at the time of removal if discussed beforehand.

This is normally followed by a course of chemotherapy, normally lasting for two to three months. Although this treatment should not affect the man's sexual performance, it may be advisable to have sperm collected and stored before treatment begins in case the treatment affects his fertility. Not all chemotherapy drugs affect the man's fertility. However, some may reduce the amount and quality of sperm. It is possible to 'bank' sperm to use at a later date by freezing sperm samples and storing them.[8]

Further investigations and treatment

If a biopsy confirms testicular cancer, further tests may be required such as a **3**
body scan, ultrasound and needle biopsies of the lymph glands to assess whether
the cancer has spread. Treatment before spread has occurred is extremely successful with a 95% cure rate.[10]

Bladder cancer

This is another cancer that mainly affects men (it is three times as common in **2**
men than in women) and can be another cause of haematuria (blood in the
urine). This cancer develops most often in people between the ages of 60 and
79 years old. If a cancer is suspected, ultrasound or X-rays of the urinary tract
with an injected contrast dye, together with a cystoscopy (using an endoscope
passed through the urethra to visualise the bladder), are usually carried out.

   About 50% of bladder cancers occur in people who smoke. Other causes **3**
include exposure to some carcinogenic agents such as aromatic compounds and
chemicals used in industry and elsewhere. As well as haematuria, men may
have symptoms such as a urinary tract infection or occasionally pain across the
pubic bone.

   If the bladder cancer is superficial, treatment is usually carried out via the
cystoscope by burning off the cancer. There may be several warty-looking
growths and treatment may need to be repeated. Anti-cancer drugs are sometimes instilled into the bladder.

   If the cancer has spread to the deeper layers of the bladder, or onto the outer
surface of the bladder, treatment is usually to remove the bladder or give
radiation treatment. Urine will then have to be diverted to an opening on the
abdominal wall and into a collection bag. Spread of the cancer to other areas of
the body is treated with chemotherapy.[11]

Male sexual problems

Men can experience sexual difficulty at any time. This might include loss of **1**
desire, ejaculating too quickly (or too slowly) or difficulty in getting and maintaining an erection. Although distressing, this will often clear up by itself and
can be helped by the man:

- reducing his alcohol consumption
- stopping smoking

- stopping the use of recreational drugs
- reducing stress
- making more time to relax.

Traditionally men are expected to be able to, and want to, have sex at all times.
However, men can be influenced by outside factors such as stress, anxiety and
illness just as women are. In fact this pressure to perform sexually can induce a
fear of failure and can in itself affect performance.

Relationship problems may also be a contributing factor and it may be that
talking through these problems with a counsellor, for example at Relate, may
help. Relate was formally known as 'marriage guidance'. The name was revised
to reflect the societal change of more individuals being in long-term relationships who might not necessarily be married. The phone number of Relate can
be found in the phone book or local libraries. There may be a waiting list
to be seen.

If the problem persists the man could seek medical help from a GUM clinic,
GP or practice nurse.

Erectile dysfunction

A man who has erectile dysfunction (ED) is unable to produce and/or maintain   **1**
an erection that is sufficient for penetrative sexual intercourse.[12] It is often
referred to as 'impotence'.

There is a great deal of stigma associated with ED which contributes to the
failure of men to seek help as they may believe that nothing can be done to help
them. The reverse is true. Interventions range from simple remedies such as lifestyle changes and medication through to more radical solutions such as surgery.

Men are often extremely reticent about admitting that they have a problem
and often only seek help after persuasion from a partner. Although the cause of
ED can be physical, psychological effects, such as the threat to the patient's
masculinity or lowering of his self-esteem, exacerbate the problem and may
even continue it after the physical cause has been dealt with.

Such patients require a knowledgeable and supportive doctor or nurse who
understands the psychological as well as the physical impact of ED on both the
patient and his partner.

Although ED is rare in men under the age of 40 years old, it can happen any
time. It may resolve without the need for any treatment.

Physical problems such as cardiovascular disease and diabetes frequently   **2**
underlie ED. Some medications can cause or contribute to ED, such as anti-
hypertensives, antidepressants, tranquillisers and recreational drugs.

Many healthy men go on having erections into extreme old age. Although there is an increase in prevalence of ED as men get older (ED occurs in 65% of men over 70 years old), it is thought that this is mostly a consequence of age-related conditions such as cardiovascular disease and diabetes rather than the ageing process itself.[12]

Managing the initial consultation sensitively is of vital importance. Read *Sexual* **3** *Health Matters in Primary Care*[12] for a clear and helpful guide to this initial consultation, investigations that should be carried out and the treatment options.

After taking the history (see Chapter 4), offer an examination. Ask if the man would prefer to be examined with a chaperone in the room. You will gain a good deal of information about how he feels about his body from his responses.

Examination may reveal a precipitating cause such as hypertension and arteriosclerosis, Parkinson's disease or breast enlargement, which is suggestive of a low testosterone level.

Investigations will be prompted by the history and examination but should usually include a fasting blood glucose to exclude or confirm diabetes. Other tests you might need to do include:

- testosterone level at 9 a.m. − low levels in the morning usually suggest hypogonadism
- serum hormone-binding globulin to calculate the free androgen index (if available)
- luteinising hormone level − a low levels suggests a pituitary problem, a raised level suggests testicular failure
- prolactin level − raised levels may be iatrogenic, or indicate a pituitary problem. A mildly raised level may not be significant. The test should be repeated as levels can be raised as a result of anxiety
- thyroid hormone and thyroid-stimulating hormone levels
- liver function tests (if drug or alcohol abuse is suspected)
- biochemical screen or full blood count (e.g. in complaints of fatigue to exclude physical illness such as leukaemia or Addison's disease)
- PSA if prostatic disease is suspected.

Treatment options[13]

- *Changing lifestyles*. Making lifestyle changes such as giving up smoking, **3** reducing alcohol consumption and taking up exercise may be all that is needed to solve the problem of ED.

- *Changing prescription medications.* Changing a patient's prescribed medication to one that does not have ED as a side-effect may solve the problem.
- *Hormone medications.* A low hormone level can be restored by medication such as testosterone patches.
- *Professional counselling.* As ED can be caused and exacerbated by psychological causes, patients may benefit from professional counselling to alleviate anxiety and stress and reduce their effects on relationships. This is often used in conjunction with other treatments to enhance their effectiveness.
- *Vacuum devices.* The use of an external vacuum device with one or more tension rings. The device is used to gain an erection by the use of a vacuum produced in a plastic cylinder and maintained by the rings at the base long enough for intercourse to take place. The ring must be removed afterwards!
- *Injection therapy.* The patient learns to self-inject medication into the side of the penis to induce an erection that can last for several hours. A test dose is usually tried in a clinic and the blood pressure checked afterwards. The nurse or doctor instructing the patient checks that the man is confident about the procedure before supplying the treatment to use at home. The same medication (alprostadil) can be used in a pellet to insert into the urethra and the penis massaged to spread the medication into the tissues.
- *Penile prosthesis.* This involves an operation to insert a device into the two sides of the penis, allowing an erection to take place at will. The device can be either semi-rigid rods or an inflatable aid. The operation removes the erectile tissue so should only be considered after all other methods have been tried unsuccessfully.
- *Surgery.* If the blood flow to the penis has been blocked either by injury or by vascular disease, it is occasionally possible to remove the blockage surgically to allow erections to occur naturally.
- *Oral therapy.* Several medications are now available, including sildenafil citrate (Viagra),[9] tadalafil, vardenafil and sublingual apomorphine. They all require sexual stimulation as an aid to producing an erection.

  Sildenafil is a phosphodiesterase type 5 (PDE-5) inhibitor and acts to increase the relaxation of the blood vessels in the penis, allowing them to fill with blood. Men who are taking nitrates, or who have a history of hypotension, stroke, myocardial infarction or severe hepatic impairment, should not take PDE-5 inhibitors. The PDE-inhibitors may interact with erythromycin, cimetidine, alpha-blockers and grapefruit juice. Tadalfil is a similar compound to sildenafil but with a prolonged action of up to 24 hours. Vardenafil is said to be more selective in action and the effects begin within 25–60 minutes, but it can be effective for up to six hours.

  Apomorphine is a dopamine agonist and is contraindicated in men who have a history of unstable angina, a recent myocardial infarction, hypotension or severe heart failure. Dopamine agonists are also used for treatment of Parkinson's disease.

Restrictions on NHS treatment for erectile dysfunction

There is a good deal of debate surrounding the medication for ED being available on the NHS. This has been compounded by the common perception that sildenafil (Viagra) is a recreational drug, and men have tried using it to enhance their sexual performance.

Unless a man had been receiving treatment for ED before 14 September 1998, he can only be given treatment paid for by the NHS if he suffers from one of a number of specified conditions. These conditions are: diabetes, multiple sclerosis, Parkinson's disease, poliomyelitis, prostate cancer, prostatectomy including transurethral prostatectomy, radical pelvic surgery, renal failure treated by dialysis or transplant, severe pelvic injury, single-gene neurological disease, spinal cord injury and spina bifida.

For other men who are caused severe distress by ED, treatment should be available in exceptional circumstances through specialist services in a hospital. Specialist evaluation varies in different regions, e.g. a specialist sexual problems clinic or as part of the outpatient services provided by a urologist.

For all other men who request treatment for ED:

- vacuum pumps can be purchased from the manufacturers
- a private prescription can be written by a doctor for injections and oral treatments. The man takes this to a pharmacist who then charges for the drug plus a dispensing charge. Charges vary and it is worth the man telephoning several pharmacies to establish the likely cost for the private prescription
- surgical treatment is provided in the private medical sector.

Further information about men's health

A useful website gives information about men's health and a list of books on men's health for health professionals: http://www.menshealthforum.org.uk.   **3**

References

1 Office of National Statistics (1997) *The Health of Adult Britain, 1841–1994*. The Stationery Office, London.
2 Secretary of State for Health (1999) *Saving Lives – Our Healthier Nation*. CM 4386. The Stationery Office, London.

3 Farmer P (1998) *Submission in Response to the 'Our Healthier Nation' Green Paper.* The Men's Health Trust, Bury St Edmunds.

4 PHLS, DHSS, and PS and ISD Collaborative Group (2002) *Sexually Transmitted Infections in the UK: new episodes seen in genito-urinary medicine clinics, 1991–2001.* PHLS, London.

5 Weller S and Davis K (2003) Condom effectiveness in reducing heterosexual HIV transmission (Cochrane Review). In: *The Cochrane Library*, Issue 1. Update Software, Oxford.

6 Jenkins J, Corrigan L and Chambers R (2003) *Infertility Matters in Healthcare.* Radcliffe Medical Press, Oxford.

7 British Medical Association and Royal Pharmaceutical Society of Great Britain (2003) *British National Formulary, No. 43.* BMA and RPS, London.

8 Clinical Effectiveness Group (2002) *Revised UK National Guidelines on Sexually Transmitted Infections and Closely Related Conditions.* Available at: www.mssvd.org.uk/CEG/ceguidelines.htm and www.agum.org.uk.

9 Jones G (ed) (2003) *Clinical Evidence* **8**. BMJ Publishing Group, London.

10 Dearnaley DP, Huddart RA and Horwich A (2001) Managing testicular cancer. *British Medical Journal* **322**: 1583–8.

11 van der Meijden APM (1998) Fortnightly review: bladder cancer. *British Medical Journal* **317**: 1366–9.

12 Wakley G and Chambers R (2002) *Sexual Health Matters in Primary Care.* Radcliffe Medical Press, Oxford.

13 Research and Development Service, Management Decision and Research Centre (2001) *Treatment Options for Male Erectile Dysfunction: a systematic review of published studies of effectiveness.* The NHS Centre for Reviews and Dissemination, University of York, has produced this abstract as part of the Database of Abstracts of Reviews of Effectiveness. DARE can be searched at http://www.york.ac.uk/inst/crd.

9

Pregnancy

Pregnancy testing and what to do with the result

Early pregnancy testing

If it is important to know as soon as possible whether someone is pregnant **1** then it is worth doing a pregnancy test on a urine sample as soon as the expected period does not arrive. The test may give a falsely negative reading in the first week after a missed period because of low hormone levels in the urine, so the woman may need to repeat it later. If the test is done very soon after ovulation, an early morning specimen may be less dilute (because of overnight concentration by the kidneys) and give a more reliable result.

The woman can buy a test from a chemist and do the test on a urine sample at home or take a sample to a chemist and pay for a test. Tests are also available free at FP clinics, advisory clinics for teenagers, some GP surgeries or sexual health clinics.

Accepting the risk of pregnancy

Many people delay pregnancy testing, hoping that the problem will go away or **2** denying that there is a problem at all. It is a common human failing to ignore problems – hoping that time will sort them out – but can have serious implications when a pregnancy is revealed at a late stage. Sometimes the delay is because the woman fears that she will be put under pressure to take an action she does not wish to take. She may be pressurised by a parent to have an abortion, or by a partner to continue with the pregnancy. In some cultures abortion is an unacceptable solution, or marriage has to follow. In some cultures or religions the man (father or partner) will assume he has the responsibility for the decision. In other cultures, the females of the family will be left to sort it out. Sometimes this will be by the mother or grandmother of a pregnant teenager taking over the care of a baby once it is born.

Pregnancy testing

A pregnancy test measures the level of a specific part of a hormone produced **2** by the placenta, human chorionic gonadotropin (HCG). The measurement is usually done on a urine sample with a strip test that gives a positive or negative value (qualitative test). The test is sometimes done on a blood sample in hospital to measure the level more exactly by immunofluorescent tests (quantitative methods).

Modern tests can detect very low levels that reduce the specificity of the test; that is, the test can occasionally be wrongly positive or negative. Levels of HCG are usually high enough to give a positive test at the time of a missed period, but about 3% of pregnant women will not have high enough levels until a week later. If the woman uses a home pregnancy test she must follow directions carefully and correctly. If there is any doubt about the result, someone experienced in using and interpreting pregnancy tests should repeat it.

Pregnancy tests usually give positive results if the pregnancy is ectopic (starting to develop in the tube from the ovary), but can give a negative test if the fertilised egg has stopped growing. In a miscarriage the fertilised egg is in the uterus but it is not developing and continuing to grow, so the test may also be negative. The fertilised egg in a miscarriage is usually lost in the menstrual flow. It may occasionally stay in the uterus (missed miscarriage) and have to be removed later. This is done under anaesthetic in a hospital as a dilatation and curettage (D&C) operation, sometimes known colloquially as a 'scrape'.

Symptoms of pregnancy

These include: **1**

- a missed period
- nausea
- inexplicable fatigue
- sore or enlarged breasts with prominent veins
- frequent urination.

These symptoms are *not* specific for pregnancy. Many women, especially young women, have normally irregular periods. These irregularities may include missed periods and other changes in the menstrual cycle. These irregularities can happen from month to month. Although pregnancy is the most common reason for missing a period, illness, travel, worry, weight change or stress can cause irregularity.

Always do a pregnancy test if these symptoms occur.

If the period is lighter than usual and there has been a risk of pregnancy

Very occasionally in early pregnancy, blood can be lost from the part of the uterus not occupied by the pregnancy. A pregnancy test is usually positive. Sometimes an ultrasound test will be done to find out if the pregnancy is continuing or whether it will be a miscarriage. Early miscarriages are very common. **1**

Ultrasound test

An ultrasound test will detect intrauterine pregnancies from quite an early stage. Transvaginal ultrasound scans will outline a pregnancy about seven days earlier than an abdominal scan will show it. With a transvaginal scan, the scanning handle is put into the vagina instead of on the abdominal wall and embryonic echoes can be detected from about 28 days from the last menstrual period. It is more difficult to define a pregnancy developing in the tube (an ectopic pregnancy) or one that has already stopped developing and will be a miscarriage. **2**

After a positive pregnancy test

A healthcare provider should find out in a non-judgemental way how the woman feels about a positive pregnancy test. It is not always obvious whether the result is welcome or not. If the woman has been trying for a pregnancy she will probably be delighted, but not always. Sometimes circumstances change and what previously seemed to be a good idea may now be unwelcome. Alternatively the woman may be initially upset, but then be pleased to find herself pregnant. Partners may have all sorts of reactions too, from indifference to horror, or from feeling pleased to being thrilled. **1**

The sooner the woman finds out that she is pregnant, the more time there is to decide on her best course of action if the pregnancy is not expected. She needs to talk to the people who will be involved and to someone who can give unbiased advice.

Unexpected pregnancy

The woman should talk to her partner — it is also his responsibility and he will have feelings about the pregnancy as well. If it is unexpected, he might not take it very well at first and be just as shocked and scared, but he will need time to think what to do as well. He might want to help and can do this by giving his partner support when she goes to talk to someone else who is unbiased.

Sometimes partners do not want to be involved, are already ex-partners or want to force their own decision on the woman. Then it is better for the woman to avoid discussing it again with that partner.

A young woman should talk to at least one of her parents as soon as she can, particularly if she lives at home with a parent or parents. She may need some support to do this from a friend, her partner, another relation or other adult. It is very difficult to cope without a parent knowing and they are usually much more supportive than the young woman expects. Even if they are not helpful, at least she will know where she stands with them. They may be upset and shocked at first, and may say things that they later regret, so advise her to give them time to decide how they can help her.

The woman should also seek unbiased advice about her options. Some advice centres give biased information designed to encourage her to make one decision rather than another, instead of putting all the options forward and letting her decide what is right for her. Some doctors and nurses have religious or ethical objections to some courses of actions when young women are pregnant, but their professional bodies require them to refer the woman to someone who does not have that belief. Good sources of help are available from most GP surgeries (it should say in the practice leaflet if the surgery does not deal with abortion, for example) and FP and sexual health clinics, and school nurses and several telephone advice lines can also direct a woman to suitable clinics.

Information about her choices can be obtained from several sources — even the BBC website has information and links to help young people decide:

- www.bbc.co.uk/so/reallife
- www.childline.org.uk and 0800 1111 (a number that does not appear on a telephone bill); also The Line, 0800 884444, for looked-after children from 3.30—9.30 p.m. (Mon—Fri) and 2—8 p.m. (Sat & Sun)
- www.netdoctor.co.uk
- www.ruthinking.co.uk

- www.brook.org.uk
- www.fpa.org.uk
- more specifically directed at termination is www.bpas.org
- more information on adoption is available from the British Agencies for Adoption and Fostering (BAAF), Skyline House, 200 Union Street, London SE1 0LX. Tel: 020 7593 2000; www.baaf.org.uk.

Making a decision about the pregnancy

The woman has three choices:

2

1 to continue with the pregnancy and keep the baby
2 to continue with the pregnancy and have the baby adopted
3 to have an abortion to end the pregnancy.

She needs to discuss all the options above with everyone involved and with an unbiased source of advice so that she has all the information she needs to make a decision that she can accept.

It is important that she is not rushed into taking a decision, but time is important too. If she takes too long, some choices, such as having an abortion or a place to live, may be much more difficult or impossible to arrange.

A list of questions can help:

- Has she all the information that she needs?
- If not, what else does she need to know?
- How does her decision make her feel?
- Does it matter to her what other people think?
- Who will give her support whatever she decides to do?
- Does she feel ready to be a parent?
- Has she thought about what she would like to be doing in two years' time?
- Does she know what is involved in looking after a baby properly?
- Has she any plans about what will happen when the baby gets older?

The woman needs to talk to someone whom she feels she can trust. If she phones to find out where to get advice, she may want to write down what she wants to say in advance, for example 'I want to talk to someone about being pregnant'. She may need to write down information like appointment times or directions, or other telephone numbers. Advise her that when a person is upset it is difficult to take in information or remember what is said, so written information to look at later is really useful.

Continuing with the pregnancy and keeping the baby

There is a lot to sort out before the baby is born and putting off the decisions for too long can restrict what is available. The woman will need to decide:

- where she and the baby are going to live
- how to support herself and the baby financially
- what she wants to do about education, training or getting a job
- who is going to look after the baby if she needs to work or do some education or training.

If the woman is still seeing the baby's father some of these decisions can be planned together. If she is in care then the local authority has a responsibility to help. If she is living at home then these matters need to be discussed with her parent(s). A social worker or the midwife can help with some of the decisions. See the section on teenage parents, p. 219.

What about the father?

Many couples will want to bring a baby up together, but unless they are **3** married the father has no automatic right to this. Whether the father lives with the mother or not, the Child Support Agency (CSA) will contact him so that he can pay towards the costs of bringing up a baby. If the father wants to share in the care of the baby but is not married to the mother, he can ask for 'parental responsibility' from the mother or from the courts. If the mother does not want the father to be involved, she will have to say why not. He will still be allowed to see the baby, unless a court decides that there is a good reason why he should not. If the mother is afraid that the father might harm her or the baby, she needs to tell the social worker or aftercare worker.

Continuing with the pregnancy and having the baby adopted

If a woman decides that she wants to continue with the pregnancy but does not **1/** thinks that she could look after the baby herself, she could consider adoption or fostering. She will need to talk to a social worker about this.

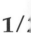

She needs to register for antenatal care with a general practice as maternity care is a separate service from general medical services provided by the GP. Not all GPs provide these services. She will be referred to a midwife who will supervise the antenatal care. Almost all care is provided or organised by the midwife unless there are complications during the pregnancy. Then a specialist such as an obstetrician at the hospital will see the woman.

If a child is fostered, the mother remains the legal parent but the responsibility for being a parent is shared with the local authority. Sometimes a member of her family, or the baby's father's family, is able to foster the baby. The child will live with someone else for a certain length of time and then a decision about the best place for the baby is reached. This might be with the mother, or it might be best to place the baby for adoption. If the mother is under 18 years of age, it is possible for both the mother and the baby to be fostered together. **3**

If the child is adopted, the birth mother will no longer be the legal parent. The adoption has to be agreed in court and cannot be changed afterwards. Although it is not usual for the birth mother to see the child again, in some circumstances, the adoptive parents will be happy for the mother to keep in touch. When adopted children are 18 years of age, they have the right to decide to contact their birth mother.

If the parents of the baby are not married, the father does not have any rights to decide what is to be done, unless he has a court order. However, by law, the social worker does have to contact the father to find out what he thinks, unless the mother feels unable to say who the father is. Children often want to know who their father is as they grow up, so it is important not to conceal this information unless absolutely necessary.

The British Agencies for Adoption and Fostering (see p. 211) publish some helpful leaflets: *Pregnant and Thinking about Adoption* and *Foster care: some questions answered.*

Having an abortion to end the pregnancy

Although people have strong views about abortion (termination of pregnancy), many women feel that this is the right choice for them when they have thought it through. The earlier the decision is taken, the less difficult it is to arrange. However, it is important to be sure that the woman has taken the decision herself and is sure about the course of action she wants to take, as a termination of pregnancy is not something that can be reversed. **1**

The woman can get advice and make arrangements for an abortion through the GP surgery, a young people's advisory clinic, a family planning or sexual health clinic. She can ring NHS Direct if she does not know where to go. If she uses an advertisement to find a clinic for advice, she should check that a full range of advice and information is available as some will only give advice about how to get support to continue the pregnancy.

She may want to pay so that treatment is quicker or carried out in a particular locality. The British Pregnancy Advisory Service (BPAS – a charitable organisation that gives pregnancy advice and carries out terminations) has a 'lo-cost' call service on 08457 30 40 30. They can direct the woman to the most convenient low-cost clinic. Marie Stopes International has clinics in some of the larger cities and has a low-cost telephone line on 0845 300 80 90.

Women can have an abortion if certain legal requirements are met. Most abortions are carried out before the pregnancy is 14 weeks' duration. It is more difficult to terminate a pregnancy after 12–14 weeks' duration. Abortions can be carried out up to 24 weeks legally, but because of uncertainties about viability (the chance of a baby living independently outside the uterus) it is very unlikely after 22 weeks.

For a legal abortion, provided that the pregnancy is under 24 weeks, two doctors must agree one of the following:

- having the baby would harm the woman's mental or physical health more than having the abortion
- having the baby would affect the health of any other children the woman has
- that the woman's life, or mental or physical health, is in danger
- there is a substantial risk that if the child were born it would suffer from such physical or mental abnormalities as to be seriously handicapped.

Occasionally it is possible legally to terminate a pregnancy at a later stage, but the requirements for this are very stringent and it is rarely considered except when the baby has such severe physical abnormalities that it is likely not to survive after delivery.

It is always better for the woman to involve the people around her if she can. It puts a lot of strain and responsibility on her if she has no support at home or from a partner or friend. However, if the woman is over 16 years of age she can consent to her own medical treatment, including an abortion. Under 16 years, the ability to consent to her own treatment requires testing against the level of understanding of that person. Generally it has to be established that the young person understands what is involved, cannot be persuaded to involve her parent(s), that her physical or mental health will suffer if it is not carried out, and that it is in her best interests to have an abortion.

Doctors and nurses have to keep information about the young person confidential and the woman should always be asked with whom she wants the information to be shared. It is usual for information about any hospital treatment to be sent to the woman's own GP. If she does not want this to happen, she needs to take the responsibility for informing the doctor about the abortion herself if necessary for any further treatment.

After an abortion, a woman may feel relieved, sad, angry or have mixed emotions. It helps to have someone to talk to about how she feels. An abortion is a very safe procedure carried out in approved premises by skilled health professionals, especially if performed early in the pregnancy. It should make no difference to the woman's ability to have a baby when she is older, unless she has a complication like an infection. She should always use reliable contraception afterwards – even if she thinks she will not have sex ever again!

Recommendations for abortion services[1]

These recommendations from the Department of Health include:

3

- the provision of support, including access to social services, for women who need more support in making their decision than can be provided in a routine clinic setting
- access to ultrasound for dating the pregnancy if there is doubt about how long the woman has been pregnant (gestation time)
- chlamydia screening
- no restriction on termination by age, gestation, income, parity or marital status
- a choice of methods of termination
- waiting times to be less than three weeks unless the clinical situation warrants it
- care for termination patients admitted to hospital should be provided, as far as is possible, separately from other gynaecological patients
- an adequate number of inpatient beds should be available for women who are unsuitable for day-case care (that is, needing to stay overnight).

Aftercare outlined in the document includes:[1]

- written information for the women that tells them when and why they might need to seek urgent medical attention afterwards
- anti-D immunisation should be offered to all rhesus-negative women
- future contraception should be discussed and supplies should be offered to everyone before discharge
- referral for further counselling should be available for those who require it and all women should be offered a follow-up appointment after two weeks.

At present, services are very variable according to the locality. Standardisation of the services offered should raise the standard of care throughout the country. It is suggested that the NHS should fund *at least* three-quarters of all abortions. The proportion is more in a few areas, but in many areas is considerably less.

In the latter, women have real problems in obtaining access to NHS provision which is often rationed to certain groups such as under 25 years or unmarried, or refused to those who are more than 12 weeks pregnant, or who have had a previous termination.

Abortion procedures

The fact that unprotected intercourse has taken place means that infection may also be present. The woman normally has swabs taken from the cervix and vagina to screen for infection, especially for the identification of chlamydia (see p. 178). Treatment should be started before the abortion to prevent infection travelling up to the uterus or fallopian tubes. Pelvic infection disease (PID) can affect fertility in the future.

    If the baby's blood group is rhesus positive, and the mother is rhesus negative, antibodies can develop that attack the blood cells of a subsequent rhesus-positive pregnancy. The mother's blood group is checked so that anti-D can be given to rhesus-negative women, and general screening for anaemia is normally carried out at the same time.

Medical termination of pregnancy (MTOP)

This method is becoming increasingly available, especially through the more specialised charitable, private or dedicated NHS clinics. In 1997, 6.6% of abortions were done by this method.

    The woman must be a non-smoker, fit and healthy, and less than 63 days from her last menstrual period. After the consultation and screening, the woman takes three tablets of mifepristone by mouth. She is able to go home and carry on as normal. Two days later she returns to the clinic or hospital and a pessary of prostaglandin is inserted into the vagina. This usually results in complete expulsion of the uterine contents within four to six hours. About 5% of women need surgical removal of remaining contents and severe cramping after the prostglandin pessary occurs in about one out of three women. Some women find the procedure distressing, others prefer to feel in control of the process and are glad to avoid a general anaesthetic.

Suction termination of pregnancy (STOP)

A suction termination of pregnancy is usually offered for a pregnancy that is under 12 weeks' gestation. It can be carried out under local cervical anaesthesia (up to about nine weeks' gestation) or under a general anaesthetic (more usual in the UK). It is usually done as a day case. The woman is admitted to hospital or licensed clinic having had nothing to eat or drink for at least six hours. After anaesthesia, the cervical canal is dilated (stretched) and vacuum aspiration removes the uterine contents. This takes about ten minutes and there should only be mild uterine cramp or discomfort. The bleeding following should be like a normal period.

Women should be warned of the possible complications as they will normally be discharged from hospital or clinic after about four hours. Heavy, prolonged or very painful bleeding, especially with a rise in temperature, may indicate infection or incomplete removal of the products of conception. Abdominal pain could suggest a perforation of the uterus (possible although rare). Arrangements for contacting medical help should be clear and preferably backed up with written information, especially if a general anaesthetic has been given. Most women feel up to carrying out their normal physical activities after 48 hours, but emotional recovery often takes longer.

Mid-trimester abortion

Mid-trimester abortions are those between 13 and 18 weeks' gestation. Physical complications after abortion increase after 15 weeks and vacuum extraction is not usually possible then.

Prostaglandin abortion

A stay of two days in hospital is usual and this may be difficult to manage in a specialised clinic some distance from home. However, a specialised clinic may offer more expertise and pleasanter surroundings. Women may encounter a resentful atmosphere in a general hospital ward, where other women are being cared for after spontaneous and regretted miscarriages, infertility or serious gynaecological conditions.

Vaginal pessaries or an intravenous infusion of prostaglandin are given and cause evacuation of the uterine contents. Most women complete this process within 12 to 20 hours and require pain relief for the crampy contractions. Following this, women have a D&C under general anaesthesia to ensure that all products of conception are removed.

Dilatation and evacuation

This procedure, carried out under general anaesthesia, is less distressing for the woman, but more difficult physically and emotionally for the surgeon and assistants. The cervical canal is dilated and the contents of the uterus removed piecemeal. Complications can include infection, failure to remove all the products of conception or perforation of the uterus. The stretching of the cervical canal can damage the cervix and increase the risk of miscarriage in subsequent pregnancies.

Abortion facts

Since it became legal in 1968, more than three million British women – about **3** four out of ten women now aged between 16 and 60 years of age – have had an abortion. The annual number of abortions in Britain (not the UK) has risen from just over 100 000 in 1971 to 163 600 in 1995, mainly because there are more women of child-bearing age but also because the procedure has become more acceptable. Nowadays, about one in five (20%) of all pregnancies ends in abortion. In 1991, nearly 90% of British abortions were carried out in the first 12 weeks of pregnancy. More than half of the women were in their twenties, while teenagers accounted for just under one-fifth. Nearly 90% had an abortion on the grounds of risk to their physical or mental health.

The number of women travelling to Britain for abortions has fallen dramatically since it has become legal in most Western countries. Of the 9300 non-resident women having an abortion in 1995, 6750 were from other parts of the British Isles (including the Irish Republic). The websites provided by BPAS and Marie Stopes International (see Appendix) give further information on abortion, including the results of opinion polls and surveys that suggest there is widespread public ignorance about abortion. Marie Stopes International has also published a report of an independent survey of women's perceptions of abortion law and practice.[2]

General information about teenage pregnancy rates

The UK has teenage birth rates that are twice as high as in Germany, three **1** times as high as in France and six times as high as in the Netherlands.

Pregnant teenagers are more likely than mothers aged 20–35 years to have low income, poor education, be unwed, be cigarette smokers and have poor nutrition. Teenage mothers and children are at higher risk of experiencing adverse health, educational, social and economic outcomes, compared to older mothers and their children.

Teenage pregnancy is both a cause and effect of inequalities in health. Teenage mothers tend to have poor antenatal care, low-birth-weight infants and higher infant mortality rates. Teenage parents tend to miss out on education and have substantially lower incomes. They are more likely to suffer from postnatal depression and relationship breakdown.

The scale of teenage pregnancy[3]

More teenage girls in the UK become pregnant than in other countries within Europe, with just over 30 conceptions per 1000 teenagers. The only other developed country with higher rates is the USA with 52 conceptions per 1000 teenagers. Sweden and the Netherlands, for example, have rates of less than seven conceptions per 1000 teenagers. **3**

Termination is the option chosen by about half of the under-16 year olds and more than a third of 16 and 17 year olds.

The latest figures (2000) from the Office of National Statistics[3] show that just over 90% of conceptions within marriage resulted in maternity compared with two-thirds of conceptions outside marriage. The number of conceptions outside marriage was 51% in 1998. Ninety per cent of teenage mothers have their babies outside marriage. Relationships started in the teenage years have at least a 50% chance of breaking down, leaving a high proportion of lone parents.

The area of most concern is the rate of conceptions to women under 16 years olds where maternal and fetal risks are highest. The death rate for babies of these teenage mothers is 60% higher than for babies of older mothers.

Teenage parents

Background information

All teenagers are not the same. Not all teenage mothers are the stigmatised lone parents living in council accommodation, supported only by benefit payments. There is a gulf of difference between an 18- or 19-year-old in a stable relationship and a scared and unrealistic 15-year-old who finds she is pregnant after unprotected intercourse at a party. **1**

There is a need for better programmes of education in sex and relationships that explore feelings and emotions as well as the factual information and the roles and responsibilities of both men and women. **2**

The information available on the outcomes of many teenage pregnancies, especially younger teenager mothers, should be more widely disseminated. Young people rarely understand about the reduced opportunities for teenage mothers to lead independent lives and to go out and have fun. Romantic views of life as a young teenage mother are best dispelled by information from those who have experienced it. The reality of looking after the constant demands of a small child, often in inadequate and cramped housing, with little money, can bring home to other young people just what they might be risking. Many of the young people who become teenage parents drop out of education. Targeted programmes can help younger teenage mothers to improve their educational and vocational qualifications so that they can become more independent.[4]

A report published by the independent Policy Studies Institute[5] provides a review of how teenage mothers think and behave during their pregnancies and after the birth of their babies. The teenage mothers came from a wide variety of educational and social backgrounds and were not the deprived group stigmatised in the popular press. Few of the teenagers expected to end up as lone parents, in council housing or dependent on social security benefits, but a year after the birth:

- half of the women were no longer in a relationship with the fathers of their babies and one-fifth had no contact with the fathers at all
- the overwhelming majority were on social security benefits with over half totally dependent on benefits
- one-third of them were in local authority housing with a further third on the waiting list.

Most of them had not planned their pregnancies. They often reported being shocked or surprised to find that they were pregnant even if they had not been using contraception. Few of them had considered termination of pregnancy. However, continuing with the pregnancy was often not so much a decision as an acceptance of what had happened, reflecting the sense of fatalism and lack of control over their lives which characterised much of their subsequent behaviour.

The babies' fathers often brought pressure on the women to continue with the pregnancy, even though the relationship foundered soon afterwards. Delight and joy at the thought of becoming a father was often very short-lived following exposure to the realities of looking after a small baby.

Nearly 50% of the women said that their own mothers had been teenage mothers themselves. Only just over half of them said that their parents were still married to each other. Half of the women had not discussed the pregnancy with their mothers at all, but of those that had, the women's mothers were often helpful and supportive. Grandparents were often shocked and disappointed, but most gave total support to the women's decisions and did not try to influence them. However, many grandparents found themselves with increasing responsibilities after the babies were born.

One of the main features of the research was the constantly changing pattern of relationships from the start of the pregnancy to the time the baby was a year old. Those who were still in a relationship with the baby's father were mainly married or cohabiting, while most of the rest were single and without a steady relationship.

Two-thirds of the women had educational qualifications, mainly at GCSE level, but one-fifth had left school at 15 years old or younger. Nearly one-third were unemployed when they became pregnant compared with nearly three-quarters at the time of the interview. Two-thirds of them said they had changed their work, study or training plans because of the pregnancy.

A quarter were receiving income support when they became pregnant compared with over 80% after the birth. There was *no* evidence to suggest that women intentionally became pregnant to get council housing or social security benefits (a commonly held myth). Most of them had known little or nothing about housing policy or benefits before becoming pregnant and the little they knew was usually wrong.

The report concludes that teenage motherhood often results in poor short-term outcomes in terms of relationship breakdown, financial hardship, dependence on benefits, lack of a social life, unexpected responsibilities, unsatisfactory housing and difficulties in forming new relationships. This research also found many young women who were happy with their babies, in stable relationships with young men who shared their responsibilities, not on benefits and living in their own accommodation. Teenage mothers should not be treated as a homogeneous group and policy and services need to be flexible to meet their differing needs.

Help for teenage parents

Sure Start schemes run by social services departments are targeted at helping young people work through the issues they need to decide. Sure Start is a scheme to coordinate help for families in greatest need through local initiatives established across the whole of the UK. Outreach workers and community projects help support families in need. Sure Start provides support for parents such as training for work and help with parenting problems.

Antenatal health and care

Teenage mothers-to-be do less well in respect of their antenatal health than older women. This is mainly because of the late presentation for the first appointment for antenatal care and because a larger number of pregnant teenagers than older mothers have risk factors for poorer antenatal health, such as a poor diet, lack of exercise and smoking. One study of pregnant teenagers reported that nearly two-thirds had smoked before pregnancy and about a half whilst being pregnant. Fewer pregnant young mothers-to-be have taken folic acid compared to those in older age groups – understandably as most did not expect to become pregnant. Young people are less likely to attend antenatal and parentcraft classes, especially those young people being cared for by the local authority.[6]

Limitations to education and a career

Some schools do not help pregnant teenagers to continue at school and exclusion often means a permanent discontinuation of education. More pressure is now being exerted on local education authorities by the government to provide full-time education for any children who are out of school for three or more weeks, which should improve the educational prospects for teenage mothers in future.

The Social Exclusion Unit report[4] emphasises how difficult life is for young mothers and partners trying to care for a child, resenting the loss of a social life and finding innumerable barriers to gaining qualifications or being able to work. Child-care costs may be prohibitively high and dependable child care can be non-existent or have a long waiting list. It can be a very isolated life, living away from their parents' home in a flat of their own, with the baby or child preventing the young parent(s) from socialising with their peers or being able to go out to work.

The Social Exclusion Unit also reports that three-quarters of 15 to 16-year-old mothers stay in their parental home, whilst around half of 17 to 18 year olds live independently. Teenage parents are likely to be housed by the local authority on large estates distant from family or other support. Some live in supported accommodation such as mother and baby hostels where there is help in adjusting to parenthood. Those young parents leaving care to live in their own flat with a young baby are particularly vulnerable to the absence of adult support and their babies are more likely to be taken into care in turn.

Depression is more common in teenage mothers and occurs in 40% within a year of giving birth. Stress from conflicts with others, worries over child care and making ends meet is common. The Association for Postnatal Illness can give support and advice on postnatal depression.[7]

The health and development of teenage mothers and their children is improved by promoting access to antenatal care, arranging support from social workers and health visitors, and by providing educational opportunities for the mother and preschool education for the child/ren.[8]

The charitable voluntary organisation Gingerbread provides help and mutual support for one-parent families.[9]

State benefit and teenage mothers

1 *Jobseekers' Allowance*. From October 1996 the Jobseekers' Allowance integrated and replaced Income Support and Unemployment Benefit for over-18 year olds. Claimants have to sign a Jobseeker's Agreement that identifies what a claimant must do to look for work.
2 *Housing benefit*. Anyone 16 years old or over on a low income can claim housing benefit – except students. Claims are made through the local authority housing department. The amount varies according to income. From October 1996 young people are entitled only to the cost of shared accommodation in the area.
3 *Disability allowances*. Disability Living and Disability Working Allowances are available to disabled people who need help with personal care and as a top-up to wages.[10]
4 *Social Fund loans*. The Social Fund can provide crisis loans in an emergency to anyone over 16 with no other money. They may also be paid for rent in advance. Budgeting loans are also available to meet one-off expenses. This is a cash-limited fund and all loans must be repaid. This fund is supposed to be a flexible system of lump sum payments to meet individual needs not covered by weekly benefit. In practice it often does not cover the need (e.g. for a fridge) and decisions are arbitrary, cash-limited and not consistent geographically.
5 *Severe hardship*. Young people under 18 years old are entitled to claim severe hardship. This means they have to be estranged from their parents, sick, disabled or have recently left care. Claiming this benefit is complex and a young person is advised to seek advice before doing so. Looked-after children (who have a higher rate of teenage pregnancy than other groups) may be eligible.

Check the current regulations – they do change quite frequently.[11]

The role of the Child Support Agency (CSA)

The Child Support Act 1991 was a very controversial piece of social policy legalisation, and can be seen as an attempt to enforce 'traditional values' as part of a political stance. The CSA requires a great deal of scrutiny and invasion of the private sphere in a marked contrast to the trend in family law. It has long been recognised that the consequences of such a radical shift in focus from a duty culture where the state looks after the children to a self-interested one has an immense impact. The state is a stakeholder in financial terms to the cost of such family breakdowns, and fears that single mothers create a new underclass and other negative stereotyping mean the state can establish a legitimate interest. The present Government has learnt from some of the mistakes of its predecessors and modified the provisions. The new law is contained in section 1 of the Child Support Pensions and Social Security Act 2000 (CSPASSA 2000), which does not repeal the CSA 1991 and CSA 1995, but makes only specific repeals and substantial amendments. Changes to the tax and benefit system mean that the CSPASSA 2000 version has more likelihood of successfully raising some children and their parent out of poverty.[12] However, the impact of the CSA on the support of teenage mothers is minimal as many of the fathers have little or no income either.

References

1 Department of Health (2003) *Effective Commissioning of Sexual Health and HIV Services.* Department of Health, London.
2 BMRB Social Research for Marie Stopes International (2002) *Women's Perceptions of Abortion Law and Practice.* Marie Stopes International, London.
3 The most recent statistics on teenage pregnancy in the UK are available from www.statistics.gov.uk.
4 Social Exclusion report available to download from the Department of Health website www.doh.gov.uk or from Teenage Pregnancy Unit, Department of Health, 5th Floor, Skipton House, 80 London Road, London SE1 6LH.
5 Allen I and Bourke Dowling S (1998) *Teenage Mothers: decisions and outcomes.* Policy Studies Institute, London.
6 Chambers R, Wakley G and Chambers S (2000) *Tackling Teenage Pregnancy: sex, culture and needs.* Radcliffe Medical Press, Oxford.
7 The Association for Postnatal Illness, tel: 020 7386 0868; www.apni.org.
8 NHS Centre for Reviews and Dissemination (1997) Preventing and reducing the adverse effects of unintended teenage pregnancies. *Effective Health Care Bulletin* **3**: 1–12.
9 Gingerbread, www.gingerbread.org.uk, or phone 020 7336 8183 to request an information pack or 0800 018 4318 for confidential advice.
10 Benefits Information Line for people with disabilities, tel: 0800 882200.
11 Information on benefits, http://www.dwp.gov.uk.
12 Information on the Child Support Agency, http://www.csa.gov.uk.

Sexual violence

Sexual violence: child sexual abuse

Underage sex

Child sexual abuse is the exploitation of anyone under the age of 16 years of age **1** for the sexual pleasure and gratification of the adult. It may be a single episode or continued over many years. It includes obscene phone calls or Internet contact, voyeurism such as watching children undress, fondling or taking porno- graphic pictures. It may include actual or attempted intercourse, rape, incest or prostitution.

It represents a betrayal of trust (that adults will care for children) and an abuse of power (that adults will act in the best interests of children). Child sexual abuse undermines the sense of self-worth that should result from proper appre- ciation of the child by the adult.

The perpetrators of child sexual abuse come from every class, occupation, **2** religious or ethnic background. Children with a disability are particularly vulner- able to abuse. The majority of abusers reported are known to the victim and are male, married and heterosexual. Women are infrequently reported as abusers, and the victims are more commonly female than male.

Changes are being proposed to the Sexual Offences Act 1956 in a bill before **3** parliament currently (published January 2003). The Sexual Offences Bill (2003) had its Third Reading on 17 June 2003. It will receive further scrutiny now in the Commons. At present the Sexual Offences Act contains two offences concerning a male who has sexual intercourse with an underage girl, even if she consents. The male may be of any age – the previous limit of 14 years of age was abolished by the Criminal Justice Act 1993. Where both are under age it is still the male who commits the offence even if he is younger than the girl, although in practice prosecutions are rare unless there is evidence of exploitation.

It is an absolute offence to have sexual intercourse with a girl under the age of 13 years. An absolute offence is one for which there is no defence that the male could have misunderstood the age of the girl. If the girl is over the age of 13 years but under the age of 16 years, a defence is allowed either that:

- he believed himself to be married to the girl and had reasonable grounds for that belief
- he believed the girl to be 16 years of age or over and had reasonable grounds for that belief. This applies only if he is aged under 24 years of age and has not previously been charged with a similar offence. (See below for changes to this age under the new proposals.)

A female can be charged with indecent assault under similar circumstances. The Crown Prosecution Service acts in the public interest, not just in the interests of an individual. However, Crown Prosecutors are expected to think carefully about the interests of the victim when deciding where the public interest lies.

Specific provisions for people with learning difficulties

In addition to the above, the Sexual Offences Act 1956 makes it an offence:

- for a man to have unlawful sexual intercourse with a woman who is a defective
- to procure a woman defective to have unlawful sexual intercourse with any man or men
- for anyone to take away a defective woman with the purpose that she shall have unlawful sexual intercourse with a man
  - *Unlawful means 'outside the bounds of matrimony'. A man is not guilty if he can show that he did not know or have any reason to suspect that the woman was a defective. This is particularly likely to occur if the man also has learning difficulties. If there is no exploitation, prosecution is very unlikely.*
- for the owner, occupier or anyone who has or acts in the management or control of any premises, to induce or knowingly suffer a woman who is defective to be on those premises for the purpose of having unlawful sexual intercourse with men or a particular man
  - *This law causes some anxiety for staff and carers of people with learning difficulties when they become sexually active. In practice, the law is there to protect people from exploitation and is usually taken to mean that the woman was on those premises only for having sexual intercourse, not, for example, if it were her home.*

It is an offence for a male member of staff to have sexual intercourse with someone in their care. There is no equivalent offence for female staff, but it might well be construed as ill-treatment or assault.

The new proposals in the bill (28 January 2003)[1] deal with the offences of rape, assault by penetration and sexual assault without consent, and causing a person to engage in sexual activity without consent. It covers child sex offences and offences involving a position of trust towards a child.

Amongst other provisions, clause 9 makes it an offence for a person aged *18 years or over* to touch a child between 13 and 15 years in a sexual way, or to intentionally cause or incite someone of this age to engage in sexual activity, unless they can show that it was reasonable to believe that the child was 16 years or over. The new bill also proposes a new offence of sexual grooming – that of preparing a child so that one of the offences in the proposed bill can be carried out. Offences against children under the age of 13 years have been extended and redefined. There is a proposal that sexual activity between someone between 16 to 18 years and between 13 to 15 years should still be an offence, but subject to lesser penalties than for someone over the age of 18 years.

The proposed bill also defines positions of trust and the offences carried out by persons in positions of trust. These include people who are in charge of looked-after children in foster or residential care, or children in young offenders institutions, schools, colleges, training centres etc.

There are many other provisions in the proposed bill, some of which are quite controversial and may be debated for some time.

Effects of child sexual abuse

Despite the rationalisations put forward by the perpetrators, the effects are damaging and often persist long term, especially if the abuse is repetitive over time and occurs within the close family (father or brother).

1/2

Survivors of sexual abuse often blame themselves. They may harm themselves or feel constantly angry. They may have difficulty forming relationships and seek relief for their feelings through drugs, alcohol, food or unemotional sexual activity. They often have low self-esteem and may suffer repeated or long-term depression. The effects may be similar to post-traumatic stress disorder with flashbacks, distress and avoidance of male contact. Many children who run away from home are the victims of abuse.

People who have been abused may have such low self-esteem that they believe themselves worthless or only valued for sex. They are vulnerable to further exploitation as adults and may become prostitutes. Others are more resilient and may be able to put their experiences behind them.

Child prostitution

When you talk to the young people involved in child prostitution they paint a bleak picture. Their parents and the care system have often failed them, leaving them feeling marginalised and disaffected. Many are notoriously difficult to deal with. Critics argue that for many of the local authorities responsible for

3

their care, bringing these children back from the brink is just too difficult and too expensive. These children exist on the margins of society – they are extremely distrustful of the police and social services. It has been described as a revolving door situation – the police hand them over to social services, but within hours they are often back on the streets. Many are addicted to drugs and they will do anything to feed their habit.

But as the authorities argue over resources, the pimps are quick to act to exploit the children ruthlessly. The human cost of ignoring the problem leaves a legacy of shattered lives. It is a tragedy for any child to become involved in prostitution. It exposes them to abuse and assault, and may even threaten their lives. It deprives them of their childhood, self-esteem and opportunities for good health, education and training. It results in their social exclusion.

Children involved in prostitution should be treated primarily as the victims of abuse, and their needs require careful assessment. They are likely to be in need of welfare services and, in many cases, protection under the Children Act 1989. Whilst there is no single route through which children become involved in prostitution, we know that the most common factors are vulnerability and low self-esteem. Vulnerable children are identified and targeted by those who abuse children through prostitution, irrespective of whether a child is living with their own family, looked after away from home or has run away. The primary law enforcement effort must be against abusers and coercers who break the law and who should be called to account for their abusive behaviour.

The Government recognises that the vast majority of children do not voluntarily enter prostitution – they are coerced, enticed or are utterly desperate. It is important that proper prevention, protection and reintegration strategies are put in place to ensure good outcomes for these children. All services must be able to recognise situations where children might be involved, or are at risk of becoming involved, in prostitution. They should treat such children as children in need, who may be suffering, or may be likely to suffer, significant harm.

The Government has issued a guidance document for the individuals and agencies such as the police, health, education and social services who work with children about whom there are concerns that they are involved in prostitution. It sets out an inter-agency approach, based on local protocols developed within the framework of *Working Together to Safeguard Children*,[2] to address this type of abuse. Its aim is to both safeguard and promote the welfare of children, and to encourage the investigation and prosecution of criminal activities by those who coerce children into, and abuse them through, prostitution.

What to do when sexual abuse is revealed

It can often take great courage to reveal what is happening. Triggers for disclosure can be concern that another younger sibling may also be abused or

1

exposure to other ways of family functioning with the realisation that what is happening is not normal. Sometimes it may be increasing age and independence. Often the abuse is not revealed until the survivor is adult.

If you suspect that abuse might be occurring but have no direct evidence, disseminating the telephone contact of Childline or the NSPCC may help someone to reveal what is happening. The Childline number (0800 1111) and that of the NSPCC (0808 800 5000) are free and do not appear on a telephone bill, so maintaining anonymity if required.

If you are the recipient of the information, it is important to listen in a non-judgemental and sympathetic manner, but without appearing shocked or horrified. You do not need to make the victim feel that they need to protect you from the horrors that have happened! A passive response to the information will help them feel that the information is bearable when divulged and help to maintain self-esteem.

You must not promise you will not tell anyone else. Explain that you have a duty to protect not just the person who is telling you about the abuse, but any others at risk, and this may involve helping the victim with informing social services or the police. Only if the abuse is in the distant past and no one else is likely to be involved (such as if the perpetrator is dead) can you promise absolute confidentiality.

If you cannot obtain the consent of the victim to follow the local guidance on sexual abuse, you still have a duty to contact the relevant authorities and you should seek the support of colleagues and/or your professional body. However, usually the decision to tell someone is a signal from the victim that they want the abuse stopped.

Reporting sexual abuse

Anyone can report their suspicions – a parent, a member of the public, a teacher, doctor or nurse. The police, NSPCC and social services all have power to investigate sexual abuse.

The social services can apply to a magistrate for:

- *an emergency protection order* if the parent refuses to allow the child to be taken to a place of safety, if necessary during the investigation. However, the law recommends that children should remain at home whenever possible, and the person suspected of the abuse should leave the home during the investigation.
- *a child assessment order* that states what kind of examination and/or tests will be carried out. It includes who will carry out the examination and where it will take place.

The investigation

A social worker will carry out the investigation. The details of any injuries, **3** the explanation for them and the abuse will be recorded. All the children in the family will be investigated.

In most cases, a doctor will examine the child. Evidence from blood or semen can be obtained up to about 72 hours after the last episode of abuse, but the sooner the better. The child should have a trusted adult with them for the examination and should be allowed to choose a male or female doctor (in theory if both are available).

The child protection conference

The social worker meets with the people involved in the investigation. Usually **2** the parents attend. The conference is required to take place within two weeks of the referral and considers what action needs to be taken in the light of what has been discovered during the investigation.

Child protection register

This lists the names of children who have been abused or who are thought to **1** be at risk of abuse (either physical, sexual or neglect). It is confidential to social and health service workers. A social worker is appointed to be responsible for keeping in touch with the family, the child's doctor and teachers, to watch over the child and give support.

It is recognised that social work departments are under-staffed and may find it **2** difficult to give the support and surveillance required. Everyone involved should be aware of their own responsibility to protect vulnerable children, and not just leave it to the social worker, but without exposing the child to multiple influences and interventions.

Myths about child sexual abuse and why they are untrue

- *It is rare.* Different studies give different rates depending on the definition of **1** abuse and the population studied, but all have found that it is common.
- *Strangers or recognisably odd people carry it out.* A close family member carries out most abuse.

- *It is so common it must be normal.* Something so damaging cannot be regarded as normal however common it is – diarrhoea and vomiting are common but it does not mean we accept them as normal. Abusers often use this argument in their defence.
- *It only happens in poor or working-class families.* Sexual abuse can occur in any family.

- *It is harmless and it can do more damage to the family to interfere.* It can be very **2** dangerous, causing real physical and mental damage. Young girls at puberty have become pregnant, STIs can be spread to children and babies have died.
- *Little girls imagine incest as part of their longing to have their father for themselves.* Freud originally wrote this as an explanation but at that time it was regarded as inconceivable that the stories could be true. A history carefully taken without any suggestions being made will often contain information that the child could not possibly have imagined, e.g. the stickiness of semen.
- *Children enjoy having sex.* They may enjoy the special attention or respond to the physical sensations if not done to induce pain. If this is the only affection that children get they will treasure it, but sexual activity is inappropriate. They are often confused by the lack of attention they receive otherwise and may behave provocatively to receive the same level of attention from adults as they have learnt to obtain by sexual activity.
- *The mother knows what is going on but does nothing to prevent it.* People find it very difficult to believe that abuse occurs. Even if the mother does realise, she may be too fearful to take action, either because of threats to herself or to the child, or to the economic viability of the family.

Working with young people

Anyone who works with young people must make a declaration that they have **1** no convictions that might prevent them from doing so. The Police Register (now computerised) will be consulted to find out if the person applying for the post (voluntary or paid) has any convictions that might put young people at risk.

Sexual violence: adults

Sexual violence information

Sexual assault and sexual abuse are crimes taken seriously by the police. **1** However, they frequently occur in the context of two people being unobserved by others, so that it can sometimes be difficult to obtain sufficient evidence to bring a prosecution. The sooner after an episode of sexual violence it is reported, the more likely it is that physical evidence can be recorded to substantiate (or refute) the allegation.

The Rape Crisis Federation was established in 1996 to provide resources and facilities to support Rape Crisis Centres across Wales and England. The federation acts as a referral service to women looking for help or support, putting them in touch with their nearest counselling service. This service is available by phoning 0115 900 3560 or on www.rapecrisis.co.uk. The service is now extended to Scotland; a list of centres is available from a link on the website.

The Samaritans (local-cost call on 08457 90 90 90) often provide support and advice for people in despair after sexual violence. Domestic violence victims can call a national number on 0870 599 5443 (Refuge National Domestic Violence helpline), or 08457 023 468 (Women's Aid National Domestic Violence helpline), all 24-hour helplines.

When violence is less severe, or threatened rather than experienced, referral for relationship counselling may prevent the situation deteriorating. Relate can be telephoned on 0845 130 40 10 for referral to the local service.

Most of the information and support available is for women. Men also suffer from sexual violence, often as part of a general assault, and find it even more difficult to admit the shame and inadequacy that follows. A contact telephone support line for men is 020 7833 3737 (Survivors UK).

Hearing about sexual violence can bring out many emotions in the listener – embarrassment, fear, confusion and often a lot of anger. The listener will often feel the same sense of uselessness and inadequacy as the victim, but it is important just to hear what is being said without trying to take control of the situation or giving directions as to what should be done next. You should have information to be able to give the person the choices that they need with accurate information.

A useful start is to read the advice for rape victims published by the Metropolitan police on their website www.met.police.uk/rape/advice.htm. This booklet tells victims how the police can help, and what happens if the assault is reported to the police. For example, it is helpful for someone to go with the victim to the police station, for the victim to take a change of clothes with them (as the clothes will be kept for testing and evidence) and never to wash before going to the police.

Someone who hears the story of a sexual assault, whether it is recent or in the distant past, needs to bear in mind what will and will not be helpful. The story may be distressing and listeners may need to be able to offload some of the emotional impact by discussing it with an impartial source of support themselves afterwards.

Do not expect a victim to get over the experience quickly – the effect may last for months or years. Accept that many people freeze when assaulted and find it impossible to fight. Without prior training, this is the usual response to attack. Do not become so visibly upset that the victim starts to feel that they have to stop talking about it in order to protect you. Often the partners or relatives of assault victims become so distressed that the victim is no longer able to mention the episode.

Listen and accept that victims tell things as they remember them − but they do not necessarily remember accurately. Respect the victim's decision on whether to report the episode to the police if they are over 16 years old. However, explaining in detail what happens when events are reported (see section above) can often help someone to come to a decision about what action to take.

Help the victim with practical things, like being checked for STIs, emergency contraception and any treatment for injuries.

About sexual violence

Like child sexual abuse, adult sexual violence occurs in all walks of life and in all cultures. Most victims know their abuser and mostly it is a man abusing a woman. Physical violence and verbal intimidation are frequent accompaniments to sexual abuse. Humiliations such as being urinated on, spat at and foul language are common. The assault may be with bottles, knives, sticks and many other objects. Some women may not have been subjected to any physical violence, but this does not make it any less terrifying.

How the victims react

Most of the information about the reaction to sexual violence is from women. Men tend to keep any episode of sexual violence more hidden. Some women will be able to struggle and scream, many become quiet and passive, especially if they have a low self-esteem from previous abuse or lack of care. If they are from a culture where they have little power, they may feel unable to protest or resist. If they have been in a relationship where the partner is very dominant, either because of personality or age, again it may be difficult to resist. Women often feel guiltier if they have not been able to resist, as though they feel that somehow this signifies assent.

Afterwards the woman has to cope with what has happened. She may be very tearful and distressed, but if she is not it does not mean that she is not upset. We have all encountered people who cannot express how they feel either because of shock or because not showing emotion is what they do in a crisis.

A sexual assault may make the woman distressed for some time afterwards. She may feel frightened, in a state of constant alertness or frequently angry.

She may have difficulty sleeping or have nightmares. She may want to eat more or not at all, or swing from good to bad moods rapidly. She may feel guilty or lose her feelings of self-worth. She may become very indecisive. She may find it impossible to allow someone else to touch her, even if she loves him or her.

Other people close to the victim may also need help and counselling. They may find it difficult to accept what has happened, blame the victim or have problems with showing affection or love.

Rape Crisis Centre help

Counselling and support are available after making contact by telephone. Some people prefer to go on having contact just by phone, others prefer to visit the centres for face-to-face counselling. The counselling is non-directional, helping the woman to come to her own decisions.

The Centre gives help and support about contacting the police, obtaining emergency contraception, pregnancy testing, STIs and abortion. Someone from the Centre can accompany the woman to the police station, hospital, clinic or court.

Victim Support

This is an organisation of trained volunteers. It can be contacted on 0845 303 0900.

If the victim has gone to the police, the police will normally contact Victim Support for them. The service will contact the victim and ask what help they need. They will:

- help with defusing the feelings about being attacked
- give practical advice and help
- accompany the victim to the police station and to court if that is required
- tell the victim about other support services
- help with the application to the Criminal Injuries and Compensation Board.

Criminal Injuries and Compensation Authority

A victim of sexual assault can claim financial compensation provided she has cooperated with the police in the investigation of the assault.

The proper form of application for this compensation is available from The Criminal Injuries Compensation Authority, Morley House, 26–30 Holborn Viaduct, London EC1A 2JQ. Tel: 020 7842 6800.

Myths about sexual violence and why they are untrue

- *Women enjoy rape.* Although we know that women can have sexual fantasies about forced sexual intercourse, the reality is not enjoyable in any way.
- *She did not struggle, so it was not rape.* Many women are so afraid that they will be hurt more, or even killed, that they do not fight.
- *Men have uncontrollable urges set off by women looking provocative.* All the evidence shows that men are able to control their 'urges' if they are likely to be discovered by other people. Most rapes are carefully planned.
- *Rape happens in dark alleys or churchyards by strangers.* Most sexual violence occurs in the home of either the woman or the attacker, and the woman knows the attacker.
- *Only young attractive women who go out late at night are attacked.* Women of all ages, classes, racial groups, cultures and lifestyles have been attacked. Sexual violence is an act of power by one person against another.
- *Women say 'no' when they mean 'yes'.* Even if a man believes this, he should not act as if the woman does not know her own mind and force her to have sex. Some women have been culturally conditioned that they should not 'want' sexual intercourse, but this is uncommon in most cultures.
- *The woman could have stopped the man if she really wanted to.* Most acts of sexual violence are planned, and the woman put into a situation where she is unable to fight off the attacker. If he is not physically stronger than her, he will use threats or ancillaries like knives or guns to overpower the woman.
- *Rape is not so bad for someone who has had more than one partner or is a prostitute.* It matters little how often sexual intercourse has occurred previously to the feelings of a woman forced to have sex as part of a violent attack on her person. This defence is often offered in court and the woman's previous sexual life is exposed as though it were relevant.
- *A boy who spends a lot of money on a girl has a right to have sex with her.* This is paying for sex with gifts – prostitution by another name – and it is still not right to force sex when it is not wanted.
- *Rape cannot happen in marriage.* Rape is a sexual act without consent; legally it is rape throughout the UK, although the law in England took some time to catch up with the law in Scotland.
- *Women make up stories about rape to excuse their behaviour.* This is rare – about the same as for other false accusations of crime (about 2%).

Police investigation of rape

The police officer that investigates the case will have received special training. **3**
The victim will also be allocated a specially trained police officer to support
them and can choose whether this is male or female. This 'chaperone officer'
will tell the victim about what is happening, contact a support group, hospital
or the victim's employer or family if this is what the victim wants, and may
help with arrangements to keep the victim safe in the future.

The account of the episode will be recorded together with a description of
the attacker.

A doctor will examine the victim, taking swabs and samples of tissue. Many
police stations now have special examination suites with a room to rest in, an
examination room and a shower room where the victim can wash and change
into other clothes after the examination. If the victim has not brought a change
of clothes, the police will normally supply some clothes to return home in. If the
victim has already changed her clothes or washed this can reduce the evidence
needed, but it will still be useful to collect the clothes and have the examination.
The doctor will also give advice about the need for STI testing, emergency
contraception and other treatment. Sometimes it is possible to have a choice
about whether the doctor is male or female, but there is a shortage of doctors
with forensic training. Any injuries will be photographed.

Other statements are usually taken later, obtaining more detail about what
happened. This is often very distressing and can take some time. If the victim is
young – less than 17 years – the statement is often recorded on video.

Going to court

The Crown Prosecution Service is responsible for taking the decision on whether **3**
the case goes to court. This is decided by:

- *Is there enough evidence for a 'realistic prospect of conviction'?* There must be
  enough evidence and it must be strong enough to stand up to questioning
  by the defence. If there is not, the case will not go to court unless a private
  prosecution is brought.
- *Is it in the public interest for this case to go to court?* There must be strong
  arguments against prosecuting, if the case is not taken to court on these
  grounds.

The first stage is heard in the Magistrates Court. The victim does not need to
attend this hearing, which is to decide if the case should go forward to the
Crown Court. The Magistrates Court also decides if the accused should be held
or released on bail. This can be a worrying time for the victim if the accused is

released on bail as they may have fears about intimidation or attack. They should tell the police about these fears.

At the Crown Court, a judge and jury hear the case. If the accused pleads not guilty, the victim will have to give evidence and be cross-examined by the barristers for the prosecution and the defence. Although it is usually distressing to have to go through all the details again, it is important to regard this as a game that the barristers are playing and not take the questions personally. The barrister for the defence has a duty to try and make the victim's evidence seem unreliable or even untrue. The victim can usually leave the court as soon as they have given evidence and been cross-examined. The Crown Witness Service can give help and support. They can arrange for the victim to visit the courtroom in advance so that it is not so strange.

It is against the law for the victim's identity to be revealed by newspapers or television.

Prostitution

Part of the culture of prostitution is often the degree of violence to which the prostitutes are exposed. They are a very vulnerable group and society tends to regard violence, and sexual violence in particular, as 'just what they might expect'.

Most adult prostitutes enter this work because of economic necessity. The low wages that many women can command, even if they can find employment, mean that prostitution can be a very attractive option. Especially in the 'higher class trade' earnings can be considerably more than most could expect to earn even with professional qualifications. So some are 'voluntary prostitutes'. Others are coerced into prostitution. They may be acquainted with people already working as prostitutes and find it easy to drift into the trade. Others are tricked or duped into it, or threatened by pimps or drug dealers.

Child prostitution is being recognised more often[3,4] and the offence of 'sexual grooming' in the proposed Sexual Offences Bill (see p. 225) is a response to the growing awareness of how young people get lured into the lifestyle. Young, vulnerable and emotionally needy young women from local authority care, or out of control of their parent(s), are sometimes coerced into prostitution during the course of their developing relationship with a new boyfriend who becomes their pimp. In some children's residential homes it has been reported that one person may become 'top dog' and use intimidation, or even force, to encourage other young people into working for her and/or for her pimp or boyfriend. Once involved in street prostitution, poverty as well as relationships with pimps or a sense of belonging to the subculture may keep her there.

Social stigma, violence, social exclusion and reduced personal safety are central to the daily experience of prostitute women as they have been throughout the documented history of prostitution. All of these closely relate to relationships with men both as clients and the controlling pimps. The lives of 'working women' are affected by our culture in which paternalistic and patriarchal attitudes still prevail with correspondingly punitive legalisation towards the women rather than their clients or pimps.

In some places, e.g. the Netherlands and Melbourne, Australia, legalised brothels **2** have been set up. These provide a much safer working environment for the women, and remove the public nuisance of kerb-crawling from the streets.

Prostitution is regarded in the UK primarily as a public nuisance. This perspec- **3** tive has influenced debates in Parliament on kerb-crawling. Regulation is based on the protection of residents and local community activists in red-light districts in partnership with the police or city council, and leaves no space for the opinions of the women working as prostitutes. There seems to be no room for a more coordinated network of services to prostitutes, playing educative and empowering roles. Outreach workers are often working on short-term projects funded by HIV prevention programmes. They are primarily trying to prevent STIs and particularly HIV transmission, but may also be able to help the women gain a sense of community and power.

By contrast, a moral position is central to the debate in relation to trafficking. Children's charities, certain feminist groups putting forward the sexual domination aspects, and religious organisations have driven these discussions. Again the voices of the prostitutes themselves are hardly heard, except as quotes in documents from the children's charities. The public nuisance aspect is less prominent in this moral debate because the practice of trafficking has so little impact on the public sphere. As a result the debates in Parliament have been shaped by non-governmental organisations rather than by local activists. The pre-eminence of the public nuisance activists in relation to prostitution debates in the UK has possibly worked to blind the public and policy makers to the extent of trafficking. Now that the seriousness of trafficking in the UK has been acknowledged, largely as a result of pressure from international organisations and children's charities within the UK, it has shaped the White Paper that preceded the publication of the proposals for the Sexual Offences Bill in January 2003 (see p. 225).

References

1 The United Kingdom Parliament (2003) *Sexual Offences Bill [HL Bill 26]*, www. publications.parliament.uk.

2 Department of Health (1999); National Assembly for Wales (2000) *Working Together to Safeguard Children.* Department of Health, London; National Assembly for Wales, Cardiff.

3 Barnardo's (1998) *Whose Daughter Next? Children abused through prostitution.* Available from Barnardo's, Tanners Lane, Barkingside, Iflord, Essex IG6 1QC.

4 Barrett D (ed) (1998) *Child Prostitution in Britain.* Children's Society, London.

Appendix

Learning resources

Books

Adler MW (1999) *ABC of Sexually Transmitted Diseases.* BMJ Publishing Group, London.

Carter Y, Moss C and Weyman A (eds) (1998) *RCGP Handbook of Sexual Health in Primary Care.* Royal College of General Practitioners, London.

Chambers R, Wakley G and Chambers S (2001) *Tackling Teenage Pregnancy: sex, culture and needs.* Radcliffe Medical Press, Oxford.

Glasier A and Gebbie A (eds) (2000) *Handbook of Family Planning and Reproductive Health Care.* Churchill Livingstone, London.

Guillebaud J (1999) *Contraception: your questions answered* (3e). Churchill Livingstone, London.

Honey P and Mumford A (1986) *Using your Learning Styles.* Peter Honey, Maidenhead.

McPherson A, Donovan C and Macfarlane A (2002) *Healthcare of Young People: promotion in primary care.* Radcliffe Medical Press, Oxford.

Tomlinson J (ed) (1999) *ABC of Sexual Health.* BMJ Publishing Group, London.

Watson E, Jenkins L, Bukach C *et al.* (2002) *Prostate Cancer Risk Management Programme: an information pack for primary care.* Department of Health, London. May be obtained from Department of Health Responseline on 08701 555 455 or doh@prolog.uk.com.

Wakley G and Chambers R (2002) *Sexual Health Matters in Primary Care.* Radcliffe Medical Press, Oxford.

Journals

Journal of Family Planning and Reproductive Health Care. ISSN 1471 1893; http://www.ffprhc.org.uk.

STI Online includes issues of *Sexually Transmitted Infections* published since 1967 and includes *Genitourinary Medicine* and the *British Journal of Venereal Diseases.* http://sti.bmjjournals.com.

Source documents

Secretary of State for Health (2000) *NHS Trusts' and Primary Care Trusts' (Sexually Transmitted Diseases) Directions 2000.* Department of Health, London.

CD-ROMs

Protection – produced by the Rural Media Company and Staffordshire University – for young people and anyone with a responsibility for young people's sexual health. Contact Kate Ryan at kjr1@staffs.ac.uk.

Other resources

Family Planning Association
2–12 Pentonville Road
London
N1 9FP

Tel: 0207 837 5432

Sex Education Forum
NCB
8 Wakley Street
London
EC1V 7QE

Tel: 0207 843 6056

Faculty of Family Planning and Reproductive Health Care
Royal College of Obstetricians and Gynaecologists
27 Sussex Place
Regent's Park
London

NW1 4RG

Genito-urinary medicine: http://www.agum.org.uk.

Useful websites

Websites often change. If you have trouble contacting any of the following, try entering the website address up to the first forward slash – sometimes the extension after that has been changed, e.g. www.womens-health.co.uk instead of www.womens-health.co.uk/pid.htm. Alternatively try searching for the words, e.g. 'pelvic inflammatory disease', by entering all the words into the 'advanced search' option of www.google.com or another search engine.

Avert (UK-based charity giving extensive AIDS information)	www.avert.org
Breast cancer	www.cancerbacup.org.uk
British Pregnancy Advice Service (BPAS): advice on and services for abortion	www.bpas.org.uk
Brook Advisory Centres for young people	www.brook.org.uk
Candidiasis	www.nlm.nih.gov/medlineplus/ candidiasis.html
Circumcision	www.circinfo.com
Cystitis	www.patient.co.uk/illness/c/ cystitis.htm
Erectile dysfunction	www.jr2.ox.ac.uk/Bandolier/band53/ b53-2.html
Faculty of Family Planning and Reproductive Health Care: journal, education and advice on contraception and reproductive health	www.ffprhc.org.uk
Family Planning Association (FPA)	www.fpa.org.uk
Genito-urinary infections	www.agum.org.uk
Genito-urinary medicine clinic list	
Genito-urinary nurses association	www.guna.org.uk
Impotence Association	www.impotence.org.uk
Incontinence	www.obgyn.net/english/gyn/ general/urogyn.htm
Infertility	www.child.org.uk
Marie Stopes International: providers of private contraceptive and abortion services	www.mariestopes.org.uk
Medical Foundation for AIDS and Sexual Health	www.medfash.org.uk

Menopause	www.the-bms.org
National Association of Nurses for Contraception and Sexual Health (NANCSH)	www.nancsh.org.uk
Ovarian cancer	http://cancerweb.ncl.ac.uk/cancernet/
Pelvic inflammatory disease	www.womens-health.co.uk/pid.htm
Prostatic disease	www.prostatitis.org
Public Health Laboratory Service (PHLS): statistics on STIs	www.phls.co.uk
Rape Crisis: advice for consumers and professionals	www.rapecrisis.co.uk
Sexual problems training	www.ipm.org.uk or www.basrt.org.uk
Sexually transmitted disease (Society of Health Advisors in Sexually Transmitted Diseases)	www.shastd.org.uk
Association to Aid the Sexual and Personal Relationships of the Disabled (SPOD)	www.spod-uk.org
Terence Higgins Trust	www.tht.org.uk
Testicular cancer	www.cancerlinksusa.com/testicular/ index.htm
Urethritis	www.agum.org.uk/ceg2002/ ngu0901c.htm
Vasectomy	http://www.netdoctor.co.uk/ sex_relationships/facts/ sterilisation_men.htm

Other useful sites

Bandolier	www.ebandolier.com
Benefits information: an A to Z of benefits	www.dwp.gov.uk
Chief Medical Officer's expert advisory group report on chlamydia	www.doh.gov.uk/chlamyd.htm
Child Support Agency	www.csa.gov.uk
Department of Health	www.doh.gov.uk/index.html
Department of Health: National Strategy for Sexual Health and HIV	www.doh.gov.uk/nshs/index.htm
Department of Health: Teenage Pregnancy Unit	www.teenagepregnancyunit.gov.uk

Gateway and Links section of the health development NHPIS site gives links to many organisations giving information on sexual health	www.hda-online.org.uk/html/nhpis
Guidelines: summaries for primary care	www.eguidelines.co.uk
Information on clinical conditions for health professionals in general practice	www.gpnotebook.co.uk
National electronic Library for Health	www.nelh.nhs.uk
National Institute for Clinical Excellence (NICE)	www.nice.org.uk
NHS Centre for Evidence-based Medicine	www.cebm.net
NHS Centre for Reviews and Dissemination	www.york.ac.uk/inst/crd/
Primary Care National Electronic Library for Health	www.nelhpc.sghms.ac.uk/index.cfm
Scottish Intercollegiate Guideline Network (SIGN) guidelines	www.sign.ac.uk

Helplines

British Pregnancy Advisory Service (BPAS)	08457 30 40 30
Brook Advisory Centres for Young People	0800 0185 023
National AIDS Helpline	0800 567 123
National Drugs Helpline	0800 77 66 00
NHS Direct	0800 22 44 88
Rape Crisis	0115 934 8474
RESPOND: for people with learning disabilities about sexual abuse issues	0808 808 070
Sexual Health Direct (formerly Contraceptive Education Service): information on contraception and sexual health for consumers and professionals	0845 310 1334, Mon–Fri, 9 a.m. to 7 p.m.
Sexwise: sexual health information for 12–18 year olds	0800 28 29 30, seven days a week 7 a.m. to midnight
THT Direct: helpline for HIV services support and information	0845 1221 200, Mon–Fri 10 a.m. to 10 p.m., weekends 12 p.m. to 6 p.m.

Other useful resources

Connexions Direct

Connexions Direct is a new service for young people aged 13–19 years that offers quick access to information and advice on a wide range of topics through one easy-to-use website.

If the young people are living in the North East, Derbyshire, Nottinghamshire, Greater Merseyside and Cheshire/Warrington areas they can also speak to a Connexions Direct advisor by telephone, webchat, email or text message. The advisors are there to listen, but can offer confidential advice and practical help too. If young people need even more specialist help, the advisors know where they can obtain it.

Connexions Direct advisors are there from 8 a.m. to 2.00 a.m., seven days a week, on:

voice on – 080 800 13 2 19
text on – 07766 4 13 2 19
web chat or email from the website www.connexions.gov.uk.

If young people want to arrange to speak to a local personal advisor face to face, then they can click on the Connexions service button on the home page for details of their local Connexions partnership. Areas covered are gradually being extended.

All advice is confidential and young people don't have to give a name and address if they don't want to. Information will not be shared with anyone outside the helpline unless advisors think that the person contacting the service or another young person is in danger or at risk of serious harm. If so, only those who need to know will find out and advisors will discuss it with the individual first and offer support.

Relate

Relate is a confidential counselling service to couples experiencing relationship difficulties. The address below can put you in touch with your local branch.

Relate
Herbert Gray College
Little Church Street
Rugby
CV21 3 AP

Tel: 01788 573 241; www.relate.org.uk.

Sexual problems

Training information for sexual problems is available from:

British Association of Sexual and Relationship Therapists,
http://www.basrt.org.uk
Institute of Psychosexual Medicine, http://www.ipm.org.uk.

Vulvodynia

Vulval Pain Society
PO Box 514
Slough
Berks
SL1 2BP

www.vul-pain.dircon.co.uk

Cancerbacup

A cancer information and counselling service. Contact:

Cancerbacup
3 Bath Place
Rivington Street
London
EC2A 3JR

Tel 0808 800 1234; www.cancerbacup.org.uk

Contraception Education Service

The Contraception Education Service provides confidential advice on contraception, sexual health and local clinics. Contact:

Family Planning Association
2–12 Pentonville Road
London
N1 9FP

Tel: 0207 837 5432; www.fpa.org.uk.

Impotence Association
PO Box 10296
London
SW17 9WH

Tel: 0208 767 7791; www.impotence.org.uk.

Index